System S

The scientific breakthrough
for lasting weight loss

System S

SALLY ANN VOAK AND
PROFESSOR ANNE DE LOOY

Michael O'Mara Books Limited

First published in Great Britain in 1998 by
Michael O'Mara Books Limited
9 Lion Yard, Tremadoc Road
London SW4 7NQ

A CIP catalogue record for this book is available from the British Library

ISBN 1-85479-325-X (PPR)

1 3 5 7 9 10 8 6 4 2

Printed and bound by Cox & Wyman, Reading

Contents

CONTENTS

Acknowledgements

Sally and Anne would like to acknowledge the following people for their invaluable help with the System S project:

Janet West, Terry Kirk and Sarah Drummond of the Centre for Nutrition and Food Research, Department of Dietetics and Nutrition, Queen Margaret College, Edinburgh; Christine Ward, State Registered Dietitian and Lecturer in Food Studies and Nutrition, who tested the recipes; Vera Churnside and her team at Fatfield, Tyne and Wear, who organised the twelve-week System S trial, and Jan Long, Sally's Assistant; Claire Ridley, State Registered Dietitian, who helped run the Fatfield study and Stephen Whybrow who analysed the data.

Authors' notes

In the diets portion sizes used are those given in the Ministry of Agriculture, Fisheries and Food book, *Food Portion Sizes*, 2nd edition, published by HMSO, 1993.

For all recipes quantities are given in both metric and imperial measures. Follow either system, but not a mixture of both. 28g = 1oz and for ease of use, measurements have been rounded off to the most convenient equivalent.

Sally
To Patrick, Danny, Tom and Mum

Anne
To Terry, Alice and Jessica

Introduction

At last – something really *new* for slimmers: a diet plan based on a sound, recent, scientific research project; a diet that's easy to stick to, that helps you to lose pounds and inches successfully and live a normal life while you are slimming; and that keeps the weight off afterwards.

Heard that kind of trumpeting before? We all have, but in this case, these claims have been *thoroughly* researched.

Over the last two years, Professor Anne de Looy and her team at the Centre for Nutrition and Food Research in the Department of Dietetics and Nutrition, at Queen Margaret College, Edinburgh, have been investigating a nutrition breakthrough which is set to revolutionise current thinking on weight loss and control.

Her discovery will, at last, help overweight people to eat the kind of foods that they really enjoy. Instead of being part of the estimated 40 per cent of the population who are overweight, they can become members of that enviable 'club', the 60 per cent who are *not* overweight.

Together with co-author Sally Ann Voak, Professor de Looy has tried out her new diet on a group of thirty volunteers in a controlled twelve-week study, which is to be published in a noted scientific journal.

This book details the fascinating story of Professor de Looy's work on this important development in the highly controversial slimming field. It also shows how the diet can work for you – with great eating programmes for people with different lifestyles, recipes, case histories and the psychological tips that will help slimmers to lose weight successfully and allow weight maintenance. You can eat out and enjoy a delicious dessert, serve up lavish, tempting meals when entertaining friends and join in when the rest of the family tuck into sweet puddings. There is

9

even a version of the diet that you can follow happily during festive occasions when most slimmers have to decide whether to avoid party fare altogether or abandon all hope of losing weight.

The goodies you will eat on the plan may seem unusual for slimmers but – as is explained in the first three chapters of the book – the choice of foods is precisely *why* the diet works. You will be asked to eat foods like sugar-coated cereals, biscuits, chocolate and slices of chilled chocolate roll, plus a huge selection of delicious meals and snacks. Drinks like beer, wine and sugar-containing soft drinks are also allowed.

It doesn't sound like a slimming diet? But then it is not just a slimming diet, it is also a weight-maintenance diet. That is what makes System S so special. The sheer variety of the foods it contains, and the way they work on your body's metabolic machinery to make *you* eat more healthily, make it the *only* diet that is really possible to live with . . . forever.

PART ONE
The Diet

CHAPTER ONE

What is System S?

Have you tried to lose weight but never managed to stick to a diet properly? If you *did* follow it, did you put all the weight on again – and possibly a lot more besides – as soon as you stopped dieting?

Are you someone with a sweet tooth, who has struggled unsuccessfully to kill your craving for sugar-containing foods and confectionery because you know they are 'bad' for you?

Do you despair of ever being able to eat 'normally' again, after years of depriving yourself of all the foods that the experts say will ruin your health?

If the answer to any of the above questions is 'yes', this book will be a revelation. Why? Because it knocks for six all the old, and many of the more recent ideas on just what kind of eating programme really does help overweight people lose weight and then stay slim.

It has been written as the result of an important scientific study which spells new hope for slimmers everywhere. The study proves that there is absolutely no need to give up sweet, sucrose-containing foods if you want to lose weight. Indeed, it can be important to eat a certain amount of sucrose in your diet because, by consuming those sweet foods, you can cut back your intake of high-calorie fatty foods almost without noticing.

Just read the comments made by real-life slimmers who have tried the diet. They were recorded during a Question and Answer session in 1996, after it was tested by our group of volunteers during a twelve-week trial held in the North-East of England.

QUESTIONER: Why has System S worked for you?

FIRST SLIMMER: For me, it worked because I could eat a lot of fruit. Other diets usually only allow two pieces of fruit. Having sweet things as well, that's helped.

SECOND SLIMMER: If you have a sweet tooth, it's perfect. You have a choice of sweet things within the diet, rather than as a 'treat', which always makes you feel guilty about eating it. The days I needed chocolate I could have it without suffering a guilt complex afterwards.

THIRD SLIMMER: She's hit the nail on the head. You don't have to feel guilty. As a chocoholic, I think this is important.

QUESTIONER: How did the others feel about that?

FOURTH SLIMMER: I looked forward to buying the different kinds of mini choc bars which are part of the plan. I used to buy a couple of different packs, and vary them.

FIFTH SLIMMER: I found it very hard to start with. I was being asked to eat sweet things that I had been 'trained' not to want. I filled up with Crunchy Nut Cornflakes. I went for quantity. I couldn't think how it could work, eating all that sweet stuff. That's been hard to accept – but it did work!

QUESTIONER: So, you had a lot of things that filled you up?

Fifth Slimmer: Yes, I ate a lot of vegetables and fruit, as well as the cornflakes. Although I don't have a sweet tooth, I need to eat a lot of chocolate at certain times of the month. I called it my 'monthly sugar cravings'. On the diet, these stopped, which I found strange.

FIRST SLIMMER: I think it is an excellent diet for anyone who hasn't been able to follow other diets that 'train' you not to eat sweet things. It is so varied and simple. You don't have to buy any special ingredients. It is easy for the family to follow. When the children had biscuits, I could join in.

SECOND SLIMMER: I liked being able to eat root vegetables like potatoes. A lot of other diets say you can't. I also eat a lot or raw vegetables, which I love.

QUESTIONER: Do you now feel differently about hunger pangs and cravings?

THIRD SLIMMER: If you follow it properly, you don't get cravings. For me, it's not so much a diet, it's more like a healthy-eating plan. It's what you know to be right, but can't usually do because you are under too much pressure to stop eating this or that food. On other diets there are always so many foods you can't have. On this diet, you can eat so much.

FOURTH SLIMMER: I feel I have been trained to eat differently. Now, I'm not interested in chips. When I was following other diets, if my husband had chips I'd pinch a few of his but now I'm not really bothered. For years and years, my friend and I have been on skimmed milk, low-fat spread and brown bread, and cut out sugar – all the things you are told to do at slimming clubs. I thought I'd be sure to lose weight, but now I don't think all that discipline really works.

FIFTH SLIMMER: Ever since I was little, I've skipped breakfast because I thought that if I didn't start eating until later in the day, I would lose weight. With this diet, I had breakfast and lost weight. It was a bonus, especially as my breakfast was a big bowl of sugar-frosted cereal. Incredible!

FIRST SLIMMER: I have lost weight very quickly with slimming clubs and put it back on again just as quickly. I was always so wary about what I had to eat, ticking boxes, and thinking about it all the time. The problems always started when I went to someone's home and felt I had to eat everything.

THIRD SLIMMER: I got fed up with diet sheets containing a whole lot of things I didn't like. With this diet, I realised that I could make up my own diet sheet of the things I really like. It suits any age and lifestyle.

Do you recognise any of the experiences described by those slimmers? Have you ever felt guilty about eating sweet foods? Or tried, unsuccessfully, to stick to a diet that banned all the foods you enjoy? Or dieted successfully for a while, then 'lost the plot' and gone back to your old 'unhealthy' eating habits? If you have, System S can help you lose weight.

(A few of our guinea pigs were not so keen on the diet, and they were honest enough to tell us why. Read their comments, the reasons why they may have found it difficult, and our explanations on pages 123–6.)

To understand how this new eating programme works, it helps to look at the history of weight-reducing diets and the modern theories that now shape our ideas on healthy eating. Even the most dedicated non–dieter must be aware that, over the last twenty years, scientists and health experts have been searching for the answer to the increasingly disturbing obesity crisis. In the Western world, we are dangerously *fat*, and getting fatter. Around 43 per cent of women and 48 per cent of men can be considered to be in the overweight and obese categories. The medical risks become very serious indeed for those who are obese – that is more than 20 per cent above their 'ideal' weight – but some of the effects increase progressively for people who are only slightly above their ideal weight. Being overweight can push up the level of fats, including cholesterol, in the blood, increasing your chance of a heart attack or stroke. It can also increase the risk of high blood pressure, diabetes, gallstones, varicose veins and menstrual abnormalities.

Many people say that the 'rot' of obesity only really set in during the post-rationing era when parents over-indulged their babies and children with the high-fat, high-sugar luxury foods that they had not been able to enjoy themselves. It is certainly true that during the Second World War the nation's diet was healthy, even though it was severely restricted in choice. We ate high-fibre, high-carbohydrate foods like bread, root vegetables and dried beans, while fatty foods like meat and butter were in short supply. No wonder that by the time the first supermarkets and junk food joints opened in the late fifties and early sixties, people were hungry for novelty foods – burgers, processed foods, TV dinners. All these were enjoyable to eat and encouraged the level of fat in our daily diets to go up.

It was during the so-called 'swinging sixties' that the amount of exercise taken decreased dramatically. People bought family cars, and drove to work instead of walking at least part of the way. They splashed out on television sets, and spent the evenings box-watching. Not surprisingly, our waistlines (and other parts!) expanded. Unfortunately, the new national 'laziness' became a part of our lifestyle; there was no going back to the old days of relying on public transport and our own two feet to get around. **Even though we started getting fatter, it didn't occur to most of us to increase our exercise levels, yet this still remains possibly the most important part of any weight-loss regime. What we all wanted (and still do!) was an easy way to lose weight.**

So, as fashions became more revealing and people struggled to remain slim, the search for a dietary solution to solve the problem of overweight started in earnest. Everyone wanted a 'quick fix' answer, and all kinds of daft slimming diets became popular. The 'Eat Fat and Grow Lean' was one common slimming diet theme; the idea was that you should eat plenty of fatty foods because they are very satisfying, and therefore your calorie intake is limited, naturally. True – except that a high-fat diet is extremely bad for your health. The Banana and Milk Diet was a favourite – just eat bananas and milk all day and you'll lose weight. The combination of these two foods does get very boring after a while, so you are very likely to restrict your daily calorie intake which is why (for some people anyway) it worked. Similar diets included The Magic Grapefruit Diet (eat a whole unsweetened grapefruit before each meal, and your taste-buds will feel so bruised that you'll be unable to eat much during the meal itself), The Mayo Clinic Diet (up to nine eggs a day, and you feel like chickening out of the whole slimming scenario!), and The Swedish Milk Diet (just drink milk mixed with glucose, and you'll lose weight or be very sick, or both). **All of these diets allow you to lose weight, but none support weight maintenance.**

The seventies brought Glam Rock, and Glam Diets, from the famous Beverley Hills Diet (eat spare-ribs, pizza and burgers one day, a selection of fruits the next and the pounds will drop off. Probably, but how impractical and how disruptive to normal eating and living), to The Model Girl Diet (steak, black coffee and hard-boiled eggs – and all the constipation you can stand!). At that time, losing weight was all about suffering – if a diet wasn't painful, it wasn't doing us good! During the same decade, one of the big 'no-nos' in dieting lore was the over-consumption of carbohydrate-containing foods like bread and potatoes. Although this has now repeatedly been disproved as a slimming theory, many people are still convinced that they should restrict these foods in order to lose weight. Food 'combining' was popular too (and has recently enjoyed a comeback), where slimmers are told to eat carbohydrate and protein foods at separate meals. The idea being that the body can only 'cope' with certain foods when they are eaten alone. This has never been shown to be scientifically valid, although the discipline involved and anti-social nature of the diet would certainly produce weight loss . . . and considerable frustration.

In 1972, a book was published which had a major effect on nutrition thinking, not only by health experts, but by the general public as well. The book, *Pure, White and Deadly*, by the eminent nutritionist Professor John Yudkin, presented convincing arguments pointing to the involvement of sugar in many diseases, including coronary heart disease and childhood obesity. It was quoted extensively in the press and had a major and lasting impact on the slimming business: sugar and sugar-containing foods were pigeon-holed as bad . . . for our health, teeth, and above all, for our figures! Since its publication, almost every diet book has recommended restricting sugar-intake very severely indeed.

The first glimmer of sanity in the whole slimming arena came in 1982, with the publication of Audrey Eyton's 'F-Plan' diet. Her high-fibre meal plans, often including jacket potatoes, wholemeal bread and pasta, helped slimmers to feel satisfied on fewer calories, thus losing weight. The meals were normal, family dishes and it was a diet that people could live with. There were just two snags with the F-Plan: some overweight people found that the huge intake of baked beans in the plan was a little anti-social (to say the least), and also doctors were worried that taking in too much bran could cause valuable minerals and vitamins to go straight down the pan! However, the 'F-Plan' did set the pattern for future diets and did encourage people to realise that semi-starvation or following a faddish diet wasn't the best way to lose weight.

In the early nineties, a whole crop of diets were published on both sides of the Atlantic which advocated eating plenty of lean meat, fish, fresh fruit and vegetables and complex carbohydrate-containing foods such as bread, potatoes, pasta and wholegrain rice. The big 'baddie' became fat, particularly the hard 'saturated' fats found in meat and dairy products, which are linked with heart disease. Indeed, some diets recommended cutting out fat almost entirely – which, yet again, led nutrition experts to worry. This time, slimmers were in danger of losing out on the fat-soluble vitamins contained in fats.

Now, at the end of the millennium, we have come to a point where people are very confused indeed as to what they should and shouldn't eat to lose weight and stay in shape. Sugar has had such a bad press that people who want to slim down are told that the 'empty calories' sweet foods contain are bound to inhibit the weight-loss process, so they should reduce it drastically. A high-fat diet is out, too, because it has been shown, without doubt, that the fatty Western diet causes all kinds of diseases, including chronic obesity. **Carbohydrate-containing foods like potato and pasta are recommended by the health experts, but there is**

still a nagging feeling among overweight people that these foods are taboo. Trying to choose a varied diet for good health these days, and lose weight as well, has become virtually impossible.

Strangely, despite all the scientific interest in obesity, and the research that has been carried out on overweight people to try and find out just why they are fat, there still hasn't been much research to find out why people are *not* overweight. It would actually be quite difficult to find one in-depth study which has really explored the eating habits of slim, fit people. Everything concentrates on the abnormal. Yet, maybe it is in the normal that the answer lies. Perhaps slim people do take more exercise and burn off more calories that way – or it could be (and this is very likely), that they simply eat similar foods to their overweight neighbours, but instinctively choose those that make them feel more satisfied.

The one 'constant' in the ongoing slimming controversy is that you *will* lose weight if you consume fewer calories than you use up. That does not mean that you should simply reduce the quantity of food and drink you consume. The ideal diet for slimmers is one which cuts calories, yet helps you eat plenty of good food to provide adequate nutrition, and leaves you feeling so satisfied that you won't pig out on the tempting fast foods that are assaulting our senses in every high street. If it can include a mechanism that actually makes you regulate your food intake and eat healthily without too much effort, it is very useful. **If it can also allow you to eat 'normally', enjoying a variety of food and drink so that you don't stand out from the crowd, it is very special indeed.**

System S satisfies all these points, including the last two. It actually does encourage you to eat the right balance of foods, almost without having to think too much about it. You can eat out, enjoying a sweet dessert instead of always having to opt for the usual 'slimmers' special' of fresh fruit or a bland water-ice; you can entertain friends with home-cooked meals which are tasty, exotic and exciting; you can drink a sensible amount of alcohol – in fact, you are encouraged not to deny yourself the types of food which are part of our culture.

What follows is a summary of just how a piece of routine research by Professor Anne de Looy, co-author of this book, became a major dieting breakthrough – the outcome of her research was a surprise . . . even to her! This is how she explains her remarkable discovery:

First, I looked at what the health education people are recommending. As almost everyone must be aware, they are advising people to reduce fat and increase carbohydrate in their diet. This makes sound nutritional sense for overweight people because, gram for gram, fat contains twice as many calories as carbohydrate. So, it is obviously better to restrict fatty foods like burgers, sausages, butter and fatty meats if you want to slim.

It is also sensible to increase the amount of carbohydrate in your diet. As a good example of the effectiveness of this, the Chinese, who have the highest carbohydrate intake in the world, are among the slimmest people on the planet. Although they also take a lot of exercise, it makes sense to assume that their diet must play an important part in keeping them slim.

Unfortunately, for Western slimmers, there is a big problem with this idea. The kind of complex carbohydrates that the experts advocate consuming, such as rice (the Chinese staple diet food), bread, potatoes and pasta, are difficult to eat in large quantities. We don't traditionally sit down to a vast plateful of rice or five slices of bread, especially when trying to reduce fat by cutting down on butter.

It seemed to me that the only way you can really encourage people to take in enough carbohydrate is to get them to top up their daily intake by adding something sweet, but not bulky, to their daily diet – such as jam, syrup, sweets or sweet yogurt. **You can then increase the total amount of carbohydrate in your diet by using a mixture of a complex carbohydrate with a simple one, sucrose. As we are surrounded by sucrose-containing foods it makes sense to use them to our advantage.**

For example, if you spread 2 level teaspoons of jam on your slice of bread, you will consume nearly as much carbohydrate as the amount contained in two slices of bread, which might be too bulky for you, and you will also avoid the awful urge to spread butter on both slices.

For slimmers, this is very important. It means that you can take any diet and reduce the total energy (calories) and still maintain carbohydrate intake by using sucrose, not as teaspoons of sugar (as sugar alone is rich in carbohydrate but not in other nutrients) but as it occurs in sweet-tasting foods.

Anne set up a series of trials to find out what happened when people were asked to add more sweet-tasting, sucrose-containing foods to their slimming diet. In the first study, she used volunteers from the Post Office.

When we encouraged people to use sweet foods as part of their daily carbohydrate intake, they maintained the total level of carbohydrate they were eating. The incredibly surprising thing was that they reduced, automatically, the amount of fat they were eating as well. At first, we thought that was quite remarkable, but when we looked back in scientific literature, studies do show that when you consume sugar or other carbohydrate-containing foods, including those containing sucrose, your fat intake falls. Could this have something to do with the fact that hunger pangs are reduced?

We put two and two together and thought that one of the reasons people might reduce the amount of fat in their diet was that they were actually cutting down their cravings for the fatty kinds of food because there was adequate carbohydrate in their diet.

In her first study of about a hundred people, including office-bound sedentary workers and those who were more active, Anne found that people could lose weight on a calorie-reduced diet that included sucrose – foods like jam, sweets, sugar-coated cereals and sweet desserts.

The second group of 'guinea pigs' studied by other researchers at the Centre for Nutrition and Food Research were an all-male group of policemen. Here, again, the sweet-eaters were more easily able to follow a low-fat diet, while those reducing sugary foods found it difficult.

The final, and most thorough test of her theory, was carried out during a twelve-week study of a group of slimmers in the village of Fatfield, Tyne and Wear, England. Sixty women volunteers took part in the study. As a control group, thirty of the volunteers followed a traditional healthy, low-calorie, low-fat, high-carbohydrate diet plan which was devised back in 1991, and which has been proved to be very successful indeed – both for those who wish to lose weight, and for those who want to maintain their weight loss. Called 'The Fatfield Diet', the plan was the subject of a best-selling book by Sally Ann Voak and also a series within a popular BBC-TV magazine programme. It is a diet which is recommended by doctors and nutritionists as one of the safest, and most effective, for overweight people.

The remaining thirty volunteers followed System S – a similar daily menu plan to the 'control' group, but with the vital addition of sucrose-containing 'Carbohydrate Boosters™': two or three sugary snacks or extras each day which raised the total amount of carbohydrate in their diet without changing the amount of energy (calories) it contained. This meant that System S has significantly more carbohydrate in it than The Fatfield Diet. They were asked to eat things like a 3cm (1in) slice of Arctic Roll (a popular chilled dessert), a 5cm (2in) wedge of jam sponge (or chocolate sponge or Battenberg cake), half a 150ml can of cola or lemonade, or 7 tablespoons of breakfast cereals such as Crunchy Nut Cornflakes, Sugar Puffs or Frosties, or 9 tablespoons of Coco Pops or Honey Smacks – **as part of their calorie-controlled diet**. Depending on the diet plan they followed (graded according to the amount of weight they had to lose and their lifestyle), they could choose two or three Carbohydrate Boosters™, **every single day!**

Not surprisingly, the thirty System S dieters were at first somewhat reluctant to follow the programme. After all, their friends were losing weight successfully on a diet with a proven track-record for success, and it didn't include sweet Carbohydrate Boosters™. They, too, wished to lose weight, so it seemed crazy to spend twelve weeks on an experimental diet which might, or might not, work. What's more, they had the additional pressure of trying to explain to loved ones and workmates that the foods they were eating really were allowed on their slimming diet plan. To be accused of 'cheating', even in fun, can be very distressing for anyone who is trying very hard indeed to fight the flab. One slimmer was frankly appalled to be told that she could eat 7 tablespoons of Crunchy Nut Cornflakes for breakfast. 'But that's unhealthy,' she protested. 'What about my teeth! What about my blood sugar level? Won't I become diabetic or hyperactive by lunchtime, if I eat all that sweet food?' In fact, no – you will find out why in Chapter Three.

There is also an additional difference: with System S, there is no huge weight loss the first week. As will also be explained in Chapter Three, this is quite normal and actually desirable. **A lot of the initial weight loss on conventional diets is actually water loss, but when you follow System S, the weight-loss pattern is much more even and steady and consists of fat – not water.** After a couple of weeks, the System S dieters found that they had actually lost a little *more* weight than their fellow slimmers. To put the (sweet!) icing on the cake, Professor de Looy's team found that the System S dieters consumed more calories overall, but took in less fat than the 'control' group. In fact, after the twelve weeks they were enjoying a healthier, more satisfying diet than their fellow slimmers, and eating such a socially acceptable range of foods that they were able to stick to it far more easily. They were eating more food (but less fat), losing more weight, enjoying normal meals and snacks with their family – and felt just great!

The study took place between September and October 1996. Since then, the progress of our System S slimmers has been monitored closely. They have continued to lose weight or maintained the weight they lost during the study. They are now used to including snacks, cereals and a whole variety of different recipe dishes in their daily diet. One of the best things about our subjects' experience as study 'guinea pigs' is that they have learned to love food and eating and no longer fear that they could at any time blow their chances of losing weight successfully by giving in to temptation. This is because the foods that tempt them the most are actually included in their daily menus. They can eat 'normally' these days. They can enjoy a sugary pudding as part of their plan when they fancy one, indulge in a bar of fudge in front of the TV without feeling guilty and add sugar when cooking popular exotic dishes. All this, without the soul-destroying 'yo-yo' dieting problems which affect so many slimmers who cut calories too low or exclude the foods (often sweet) which they really love.

You can read revealing case histories from six of the thirty volunteers in Chapter Seven. There is no doubt that System S has proved to have been very effective indeed for real-life slimmers, especially for those who have a sweet tooth, or who have tried, unsuccessfully, to lose weight on other diets.

System S helps slimmers to lose weight by helping to control their appetite while making them feel that life is actually worth living. Once you try it, you will find that you can eat a wide variety of foods, and go on enjoying your favourite foods as part of your diet for the rest of your life. Like any other weight-reducing diet, it is not suitable for growing children.

Six Steps to System S

Here is a summary of the six facts that explain the scientific theory that makes the System S Diet so special.

1. To shed weight, you must consume less energy, in the form of calories, than you expend. So, if you are currently eating foods containing about 2500 Cals every day and you are gradually gaining weight, you could reduce your calorie intake to about 1500 and lose weight safely.

2. The current healthy eating message from experts is to eat less fat – and more carbohydrate-containing foods – bread, potato, pasta. That means balancing your daily calorie intake so that less than 35 per cent of your day's calories comes from fat and at least 50 per cent from carbohydrate.

3. This makes sense for slimmers because, gram for gram, carbohydrate contains less than half the calories of fat. For instance, a 28g (1oz) portion of butter contains 210 Cals, while a 28g (1oz) slice of wholemeal bread contains only 61 Cals.

4. Increasing the amount of carbohydrate in ordinary meals is obviously the best way to slim. In an ideal world, you would be able to do this, but in our culture it is difficult. You do not normally sit down to a plateful of plainly boiled rice at every meal, a huge portion of spaghetti or four slices of bread. If you do consume vast quantities of these foods without adding extra fat in the form of sauces or spreads, you will find them very difficult to eat. What's more, favourite mealtime basics like cheese, meat, eggs and fish contain fat, but either no carbohydrate at all, or very little, so they don't help 'bump up' your carbohydrate intake.

5. Adding a simple carbohydrate – sucrose – can top up your total carbohydrate levels in an easy, palatable way, without adding too many calories. For instance, if you spread 2 level teaspoons of strawberry jam on your slice of wholemeal bread you will add 10g of carbohydrate but only 40 Cals. This is a far more enjoyable and tasty way of getting extra carbohydrate than adding an extra slice of bread. Even if you ate it dry, you would add at least 60 Cals to your daily total, and the same amount of carbohydrate – just 10g. If you added butter as well, you could bump up the calorie total to 100.

6. If you do consume enough carbohydrate in your diet, you will cut down on fat with very little effort. Put simply, if your carbohydrate intake for the last few days has been adequate, when you sit down to supper tonight you will be less likely to want those greasy chips or to smear butter all over your slice of bread. (On page 129, find out how successful slimmer Muriel Farr stopped craving fatty 'extras' like cheese on the top of her soup and butter on bread and potatoes, once she had been following System S for just a few days.)

This breakthrough means that you can – and indeed, should – eat some sweet foods every day, plus a wide variety of foods like lean meat, fish, fruit, vegetables, pasta and cereals, and a little alcohol if you want it. We now know that cutting out all sugar-containing foods is unrealistic in our society today and not a good idea, just as it is not good for your health to cut all fat out of your diet.

Waist Measurement Chart

Here's a simple way to find out if you need to lose weight. Simply measure your waist at its narrowest point and check the comments below:

Women

Less than 80cm (31½in): You are within the desirable range. If you want to lose a few pounds with System S, the Basic, Easy Cook, Vegetarian or Sport and Fitness Plans will probably suit you best, and exercise will help you tone up.

Between 80cm and 88cm (31½in and 34½in): You should lose some weight – the Steady, Gourmet, Easy Cook or Vegetarian plans are all suitable. Start a gentle exercise plan, working up to a more demanding routine.

Over 88cm (34½in): You should take immediate action to shed weight. Go for the Steady, Gourmet or Vegetarian plans, gradually increase the amount of exercise you take and check with your doctor before embarking on any diet or fitness plan.

Men

Less than 94cm (37in): You are within the desirable range. To lose a few pounds, choose the Active Man, Vegetarian or Sport and Fitness plans and combine them with a regular exercise routine.

Between 94cm and 102cm (37in and 40in): Action is needed! Active Man, Gourmet, Vegetarian or Sport and Fitness Plans will all suit you. And don't forget the exercise.

Over 102cm (40in): Take action now! Go for the Gourmet, Easy Cook, Vegetarian or Steady Plans and take some gentle exercise. Have a medical check-up before you start.

CHAPTER TWO

The Scientific Bit!

This chapter helps you to understand the scientific reasoning behind System S. In it, Professor Anne de Looy explains why the diet is put together in the way it is, and answers many of the questions slimmers ask. As she so wisely admits, there are simply *no* answers to some of the questions, despite all the research carried out by scientists. She writes: 'Why some people become overweight, and then obese, is still largely a mystery although, in scientific terms, the explanation is very simple and straightforward. An overweight person has taken in more energy (calories) than is needed, and the body, being very cautious, has decided to save the energy for times when the food supply is scarce. It is something that can happen to anyone at any time, and don't let people fool you that it can't!'

What is infuriating to you if you are trying to lose weight is that you are bound to know different people who can apparently eat the same amount as you and yet put on widely different amounts of extra fat (in some cases, apparently no fat at all!). This variation has a lot to do with who you are and how your lifestyle operates.

This is very difficult to study and it is impossible to judge the way a person uses energy just by looking at them. For example, if you measured how many calories two people use up while asleep you could find that one person used one and a half times as many as the other. Yes, incredibly, this measurement has been done by scientists. So, you see, if one person uses more energy while they are asleep, this could easily account for why they seem to eat more and do not become overweight. Of course, there may be other explanations as well. They could take more exercise, have a very active job or use extra energy because they are nervous, 'twitchy' individuals who cannot relax and sit still. Whatever the explanation, the same simple equation still holds good: if the amount of energy (calories) you take in is the same as the amount you use, then you will not store any fat. If you eat more than you need, you will store the extra as fat; if you eat less than you need, you will lose fat and grow slimmer. Simple isn't it?

Yet, if it is so simple, why is it that some people living in the same family, in the same road, in the same city or working in the same office do not become overweight or obese, while others do? There are really no answers to these questions, but there are glimmers of answers and that is what this chapter is all about. As well as explaining how and why System S works, it will help you to understand yourself which, in turn, will make you more successful in losing weight and – most important of all – in keeping it off.

Living in the Real World

Although many things are involved, there is one basic factor which applies to us all: whether you find it easy or difficult to lose weight probably starts with your parents – bless them! None of us can do anything to change that situation.

Much research has been done to show that not only do you inherit the colour of your eyes, your wonky nose or extra-large feet from your mum or dad, but other characteristics as well such as your metabolism – the way your body deals with the 'fuel' that you put into it. This means that you may be more efficient than your brother or sister at handling the energy that comes into your body. If you are a food lover, this is bad news because it means that you can probably get by on less food, and therefore any extra food that you put in your mouth is likely to be stored as fat. However, the news isn't all bad, because at least you know that you can make a decision about your eating habits. You can change the composition of your diet, eating fewer fatty foods, which provide more calories weight for weight, in order to counteract nature's unfair 'whammy', and maintain a healthy weight.

It must be stressed that the way you put on (or do not put on) weight is very unlikely to be anything to do with 'hormones' or 'heavy bones'; it is to do with how your body uses its energy. **Although there is a wealth of evidence building up which points to the importance of what you inherit from your parents, there is also another factor at work: the food culture or environment you find most comfortable.** During our System S researches in Fatfield, we had one family who enjoyed home baking and cooking in general. Not surprisingly, mother and daughter found it very difficult to control their weight. Their food environment and culture was hardly of help. So, here is a question which you must consider when you are trying to slim – how well does your food culture help or frustrate your efforts at food control?

Interestingly, other research has shown that some of us develop a specific psychological pattern to help us deal with our food culture. These patterns can be tested for scientifically by a psychologist, but I am sure that most of us can recognise them in ourselves without needing to take a test. For example, you may be an 'inhibited' eater. This type of person is so concerned about what they are eating that they control their food intake all the time, sometimes successfully and sometimes not. The people who are most likely to be 'inhibited' are those who have reduced their body fat on a diet, and are maintaining that weight loss, but are perpetually worried about piling on the pounds again. Some people deny this state of mind, but it is a well-recognised syndrome and it can be damaging to your long-term health. Put simply, it's the 'I've-blown-it-already-so-I-might-as-well-stuff-myself' pattern. Do you recognise this in yourself? You have one chocolate biscuit, and then, because you've broken your diet you go on to eat the whole packet. Other research has shown that 'inhibited' eaters are likely to eat more when they are in company with others who are overeating or when they know that they will be going somewhere where lots of food is available.

On the other hand, 'non-inhibited' eaters do not alter their food intake when the environment around them changes. They seem to be more in control of their food intake and appetite.

In experiments with 'inhibited' and 'non-inhibited' eaters, both kinds of eater were given a milkshake and then asked to taste some other foods. The 'inhibited' eaters always ate more than the 'non-inhibited' eaters, having become disinhibited by wolfing down the milkshake. It is as if they feel they have already eaten one thing, so they might as well go on and finish the job. However, in the same experiment, the 'non-inhibited' eaters ate the same amount of food afterwards whether they had had a shake or not. This is sometimes referred to as 'internal control': the 'non-inhibited' person being much more in control of themselves and not letting external events control their food intake.

So, if you recognise yourself as an 'inhibited' eater, what can you do about it? Well, recognising this pattern is the first important step and the second is to find lots of support by talking it through with diet counsellors and other dieters who can give you tips on how to come to terms with this type of eating. Sadly, diet counselling is not always readily available, but it is worth having a chat with your doctor who can put you in touch with any recommended counsellors in your area. They could be attached to your hospital, within a well-run healthy eating group, or even within the medical practice itself. Many surgeries now have experts on hand who can help you.

If you have this problem, it is important to know two things. The first is that individual foods *in themselves* are not bad or good for you. It is the amount you eat and the combination of foods you put together over days, weeks and months which may prevent you from realising your personal goals. For example, tucking into fish and chips once a week is not going to make you gain an additional pound in a week. However, if you eat a fish supper *every day* in addition to the rest of your food, or always finish off with spotted dick and custard, then you are likely to gain weight. (Finishing off a fish supper with a pudding is, of course, typical disinhibited eating behaviour because you know you should not be having it, whereas the 'non-inhibited' eater wouldn't worry.)

The second important fact is that some foods look more calorific than they are – they have fewer calories in them than you might think from their size on the plate. For example, a sausage roll has about 300 Cals, but a roasted chicken drumstick, bigger than the sausage roll, has only about 150 Cals. A piece of fruit cake has about 400 Cals, yet a large chocolate eclair with whipped cream has about 200 Cals. In comparing different food items, **the size of the food is no indication of the calorific value.** Choosing small does not mean you are automatically choosing fewer calories.

You should learn to love the foods you eat; to savour and gorge on low-calorie foods as part of your diet will give you lots of value with a lower calorie intake. You are in control. **You should not worry about including foods in your diet such as fish and chips, burgers or pizza when you are confident that you want to eat them, and not because you are feeling guilty about breaking your diet.** Make sure you include those foods *you know* are calorific *as part* of your diet and *not additional* to it. Many lean people eat burgers and pizza without feeling guilty: can you do the same as part of your diet? Can food in your life take on a new culture?

Here is a little story: when my children were small, my husband and I used to go into raptures about raisins and carrots in front of them. We told them that if they were very good they could have treats of carrots and raisins. Of course, they grew up thinking that these were really important 'treat' foods until they met chocolate at school. When we moved to Scotland from Yorkshire, I sent the children to school with carrots in their packed lunch boxes. Much to my amazement, my youngest daughter came home one day saying she had swapped her carrots for sweets. Evidently, other children prized the carrots over their sweets. This is an interesting and serious example of a food culture. **Treats are what we make them. All food can be treats, even carrots if we want them to be.** The interesting psychology here is the role of other people in defining 'treats', especially those in the advertising industry. Some manufacturers tell you that certain treats are really naughty (but nice!), so when we eat them we are made to feel guilty as part of the treat experience! This type of psychological selling is a complete disaster for 'inhibited' eaters.

In System S, we have made sweet foods important, not because we want you to think of them as treats but because we need to live with these foods every day, and we want you to feel comfortable with them; learn to be 'in control' and live in the real world. The other fascinating reason is because these very foods – normally considered taboo for slimmers – can actually help you control your appetite.

Appetite Control

There has been interesting research carried out on what controls our appetite for food, and especially on what makes us stop eating a particular food. We have already discovered that there are psychological influences at work here, but there is also an effect from the type of foods we eat.

We know that our food is made up of proteins, fats and carbohydrates and of course we also use alcohol as a 'food'. The body stores protein only as part of muscle tissue and it stores a very small amount of carbohydrate as glycogen. Sensibly, it doesn't store alcohol at all because it is a body poison. The body regulates the amount of these substances eaten by us through control of our appetite. However, when it comes to fat, the body is not very good at controlling the amount we eat. As we know only too well, fat can be stored in what seems to be unlimited quantities! If that wasn't bad enough, research has also shown that people who are overweight or obese actually use fat in a different way from lean people. It has been suggested that some people cannot burn fat in the body as easily as others, and both overweight and lean 'inhibited' eaters show this tendency. This means that when they do eat fat then they are more likely to store it than their leaner friends.

There are two important messages for us here:
- *We must be careful how much fat we actually put into our mouths.*
- *We have to be aware that some people may handle fat differently in their bodies.*

What does research have to say about these two aspects? Well, if you look at what overweight and obese people are eating, you will find that they tend to have more fat in their diets than lean individuals. They also tend to have less carbohydrate because wherever you find a highish fat intake, you tend to find a low intake of carbohydrate. Now, if the body has a low carbohydrate intake and the body's store is controlled by appetite, then you are much more likely to crave more carbohydrate. The result is hunger!

There is also another angle to this story. During an experiment, some people were given a high-carbohydrate drink, and others a high-fat drink and were then asked how hungry they were a certain time afterwards. The high-carbohydrate drink caused less hunger. People were still hungry after they had sipped a high-fat drink. **So, it seems that high carbohydrate intake reduces appetite far more successfully than high fat intake.** Very recent results from research on people who have lost weight successfully shows that their weight-maintenance diet tended to be high in carbohydrate and low in fat; they seem to have learned the secret of success in keeping the weight off.

Sugar is a carbohydrate. In any diet there is a relationship between fat and sugar. The less fat people consume, the more sugar they absorb. This is sometimes referred to as the fat–sugar see-saw. Sugar, as we all know, makes food tasty. It is not at all bulky; by that I mean that there is the same amount of carbohydrate in 2 teaspoons of sugar as there is in a thin slice of bread or a small jacket potato. But sugar on its own has no additional nutrients, so you need to eat it as part of another food. Bread, potato, pasta and rice are more bulky and they are thought of as very good and nutritious parts of our diet. They should be eaten in quantity because, being very good sources of carbohydrate, they can help us control our appetites. The only trouble with this form of carbohydrate is that it may be difficult to eat in the bulk required. We often want to put fat on our potatoes or bread and it is difficult to snack on potatoes, rice and so on. So, it seems sensible to use sugary foods as part of your carbohydrate supply and these are easily available as snack foods and generally very much part of our food culture. This is the basis for introducing Carbohydrate Boosters™ as part of System S. A full list of these is given in Chapter Four (pages 61–2). We want you to get used to the idea of using these previously 'forbidden' foods as part of your diet so that you can learn to see them, not as 'baddies' but as part of your normal, and indeed anyone's, normal, food pattern.

One additional note of interest. You may well be thinking that fat is often associated with sugar, for example in chocolate and cakes. Again, scientific research has come up with some interesting findings. As we have already seen, overweight and obese people have a definite preference for fatty food, which is why their diets are often high in fat. But, laboratory tests have found that it is the fatty food associated with savoury and salty tastes (e.g. crisps, nuts or chips) which were preferred, *not* the fatty sweet foods like cakes or pastries. While studies of groups of people have found that high-fat diets are linked with being overweight and obese, there is no link between sugar and excess weight.

There are many good reasons for reducing the fat in your diet, but we prefer to follow a more positive message: *increase* the carbohydrate in your calorie-reduced diet to suit your metabolism and your health. This is the successful formula for System S.

Lifestyle

At the beginning of this chapter, I talked about the importance of eating fewer than the total amount of calories you need every day in order to lose body weight. There are many good medical reasons why reducing your body weight is important, such as cutting the risk of heart disease, hip or other joint replacement and reducing high blood pressure. One thing which will help you increase the amount of calories you burn every day and reduce the risk of illness is *exercise*.

By talking about exercise, I don't necessarily mean going to the gym, cycling or jogging for long distances. Any gentle exercise, if done regularly and over a long period, will help you to lose weight more quickly and make you fitter. **Many of our System S 'guinea pigs' felt so much better on their diet and were so encouraged that they engaged in more activities.** A favourite was swimming. So, making a change to your lifestyle in this way is to be recommended. It is also interesting to know that not only does exercise help with weight loss, but it also gives you an extra 'buzz' once started. System S principles are strongly recommended for those who intend to work up their exercise abilities to a slightly higher level as well. Adequate carbohydrate is very important for any athelete or sportsperson, and the diet provides plenty. A special version of the diet in Chapter Six (see page 108) will help anyone who wants to train for a fun-run, tennis match or swimathon.

How will your lifestyle be different with System S?

First, you can enjoy the types of food which are part of all our lives. Yes, you will need to be careful what you eat, but you can feel part of the family and part of society. As real-life slimmers relate in Chapter Seven, this takes some getting used to and other members of your family and friends may find it difficult to believe. They are still thinking that certain foods are 'bad', 'naughty' or 'sinful'. *You* know that all foods are potentially good or bad depending on how you choose to use them. Changing your lifestyle to be someone who doesn't need to be different is a challenge but one we think you can rise to.

Second, the best recipe for keeping weight off is to learn to like carbohydrate and reduce fat (remember the research that seems to indicate that successful weight-losers have changed their diet to high carbohydrate and low fat?). System S positively encourages you to change your eating habits or food culture . . . or both. This means being aware that there are outside forces, particularly in the advertising and food retail industries which could confuse the issue by giving you conflicting messages about what you should, or shouldn't, eat on a healthy diet. We now have many low-fat products on the market. Unfortunately, they are often low-sugar as well – so they will not help you to control your appetite. **Remember, you need to have sufficient Carbohydrate Boosters™ within your System S diet plan.** That means two, or even three every single day. If you don't do this, then you will be more hungry than you should be. Similarly, don't forget to snack.

This diet may seem unusual, even revolutionary, but it falls into line with all current government recommendations concerning health. It is low in fat, high in carbohydrate and also helps you lose weight and remain slim. In this book, we give you a taste of this way of eating. We could advise you to start off your meal by eating your dessert, and working backwards towards the fish or meat, but for most people (and their families) this would be difficult. So, we encourage you to eat more healthily by planning meals which do not seem particularly unusual although they *are*. As you learn to enjoy this way of eating – and realise that it can help you lose weight and stay slim – you will want to devise your own high-carbohydrate menus. The recipe section at the back of the book (pages 139–88) will give you a good start.

The scientific basis for the diet has been explained and hopefully you have found it convincing. But successful diets are about people as well as theories and scientific studies. So the last thing we did on System S was to ask people some questions about their attitudes and beliefs towards dieting before they started the diet. These questions were not specifically about System S, in fact they had no idea what diet they would be following. We wanted to see if their ideas would change over the course of the twelve-week study, and whether there were any important differences between the motivation of the various people on the diet.

What we found was (and it will come as no surprise to most slimmers!) that those who thought they would have little chance of following the diet successfully were the people who dropped out of the trial very early. Right from the start, they believed that they would not do well. We also found that those people who thought they would be able to reduce the amount of fried or fatty foods they consumed did well. Interestingly, so did those who said that they could reduce the amount of sweet foods in their diet (although they later found out that they didn't have to!). **What these people were telling us was that they were ready to diet and had the right attitudes and beliefs about their ability to succeed.**

This is very important. If you believe you are not yet ready for dieting, then *any diet* will fail. We have to have a strong belief in ourselves to ensure success. Research has shown that whenever we have a major life change such as giving up smoking or taking

CHAPTER THREE

Exploding the Myths

Picture any motorway restaurant. A family – mum, dad (who is very overweight) and two small children – sit at a café table, with a meal in front of them. The meal is a typical fast food spread: burgers, onion rings in batter and french fries. Also on the table is a bag of sweets. Sneakily, one of the children stretches out a hand and takes a sweet, popping it into his mouth quickly. Dad looks up from his half-eaten burger, pile of greasy onion rings and chips and says: 'All right, son, but just one – you'll be fat like me if you get a taste for sweets.'

This scene illustrates perfectly the taboo that surrounds the consumption of sweet things in most Western countries. No matter that the meal the family is eating is fat-loaded, and a recipe for a heart attack – sweets are the villains!

Right from early childhood, we are brainwashed into believing that sweets, chocs, puds, cakes and biscuits are all *bad*. Of course they are, if they are consumed in quantity at the expense of other foods. Unfortunately, the more you ban something, the greater the desire for it. That is one of the reasons why so many overweight people have a very difficult relationship with confectionery, chocolate and other sweet foods, and why the consumption of all these is so high.

If you've ever sneaked a choc bar into your supermarket trolley, or hidden a whole cache of sweets in your car, bedroom or schoolbag, you will know that the feeling of guilt surrounding sweet-eating is almost drug-like: you hate yourself for doing it, yet do it again and again. Then, when you want to lose some weight, the first thing you feel you must cut out completely are the sweet snacks that give you the most pleasure.

That is when your problems start. For when sugar is eaten in moderation and in combination with other carbohydrate-containing foods like bread and potatoes, it gives a feeling of 'satiety' – that is, it fills you up (see Chapter Two). Once you stop eating enough carbohydrate you will get hunger pangs which must be satisfied, and you will crave food, often high-fat items like chips and takeaways, which are calorie-loaded.

When you follow System S, you must eat some sweet foods every single day. The sucrose is in the form of a Carbohydrate ('Carb' for short) Booster™ – a snack which can be nibbled whenever you like. You'll need several of these each day on the diet – the number will vary according to your diet choice (see Chapter Five). They can be eaten at any time, to suit you. The golden rule is: *never forget to have your Carb Boosters™*!

As was mentioned in Chapter One, some of the System S 'guinea pigs' found it difficult to eat the Carb Boosters™, not because they didn't fancy a slice of cake or a portion of ice cream but because they, like most of us, have been conditioned to believe that these foods contain just 'empty calories' and are bad for slimmers. They even experienced a lot of criticism at home and work when they ate their Boosters™ in front of other people. 'I was often teased by my husband for nibbling my chocolate bars and sweets,' says housewife Deborah Handy, who tells her story on page 130, 'But, as soon as he noticed that I was losing weight steadily, the teasing stopped.'

Here is a list of common assumptions – plus the real facts – about eating sugary foods. Read it carefully and you will see that, when it comes to losing weight and keeping it off, sugary foods are certainly not the villains that they have been made out to be.

Ten Common Assumptions about Sweet Foods

1. Sweet Treats Make You Fat

It's true that eating too much of anything will make you put on weight, but sweet foods are not necessarily more calorific than those without sugar. In fact, a sweet snack can be much lower in calories than a high-fat, savoury one. For instance, a mini-size choc bar contains about 100 Cals, while a 50g (2oz) piece of Cheddar cheese would 'cost' about 230 Cals . . . more than double. A fruit yogurt has a modest amount of calories (about 150 per carton), compared with a bag of chips (about 350 Cals). Many breakfast cereals containing sugar are not substantially higher in calorie-content than the no-sugar 'slimmers' cereals. **Kelloggs sweet-tasting Coco Pops have only 108 Cals per 25g (1oz), which is a mere 3 calories more than Special K, the popular Kellogg's brand which actually targets shape-watchers in a series of highly successful television advertising campaigns.**

2. Eating Sweets Is Addictive

Many slimmers are so frightened of their sweet 'addiction' that they avoid any contact with sweet foods, even to the point of not going near a sweet shop or keeping a box of chocolates in the house. They argue that if they eat just one sweet item, they will be 'biologically programmed' to want more and more. Certainly, this can happen if you let yourself become so hungry that your blood sugar level falls and you crave a sugar 'fix'. If there is a packet of biscuits or box of chocs around, you will obviously feel inclined to scoff the lot. On the other hand, if you eat regular, balanced meals (like the System S meals), you will feel full and satisfied and the hunger pangs are less likely to hit you just when you happen to be outside a sweet shop! As far as the biological effects of certain foods are concerned, scientists now believe that there is no physiological reason why people do experience cravings for specific foods. What the most-craved foods (such as sweets and chocolates) appear to have most closely in common is their role as 'nice but naughty' treats. In other words, the more you think you won't have any control over your desire for sweets, the more likely you are to pig out. So, it's much better to indulge your fancy for something sweet every day than to work yourself up into a lather of guilt and indecision while you try to avoid temptation.

3. Sweets Are Bad for Your Teeth

Although it is true that sugar is a factor in the dental decay process, all types of sugars, including those in fruit, can feed the plaque bacteria which cause decay. Even starch, especially when it is highly processed, can promote decay in the right conditions. This is because it is broken down into sugars in the mouth. Research has found that the level of sugar in a food is less important than how quickly the food is cleared from the mouth. In other words, whatever you eat or drink, it is vital to brush and floss teeth properly after eating, and use a toothpaste containing fluoride. Remember, too, that brushing *before* you eat is a good way of removing the plaque that attracts sugars.

Unless you normally suck sweets all day long and never clean your teeth, simply reducing the sweet foods in your diet won't make a jot of difference to your dental health. For children, the rule is that eating sweets is fine, in moderation and after meals, so long as they eat plenty of other foods as well, and clean their teeth regularly. Nowadays, the message is simple: whatever you eat or drink, you must brush and floss properly. Luckily, this message is getting through. Thanks to better dental habits and fluoridation of water, England and Wales have one of the lowest levels of tooth decay in Europe, despite a high level of sugar consumption.

4. Sugar Is just 'Empty' Calories

If you put 4 teaspoons of sugar in your tea, you'll add 68 Cals. If you do that six times a day, the calorie total adds up to a substantial 408 Cals. The only nutrient supplied will be sucrose – a simple carbohydrate. If you are trying to lose weight and stick within a daily calorie total of about 1500, those calories could be better spent on something more nutritious. Four hundred Cals is enough for a good meal which could include rice or pasta, fruit, fresh fish or lean meat, vegetables and a sweet dessert.

However, if you look at foods which contain sugar plus other nutrients, you get a very different picture. For instance, low-fat fruit yogurt has sugar (i.e. sucrose), protein and calcium, for growth and healthy bones. A slice of wholemeal bread spread with jam is a sweet treat which includes sucrose, fibre, Vitamins B, C and E and calcium; so, it can hardly be described as 'empty'. In the dietary studies carried out at the Centre for Nutrition and Food Research for System S it was found that sucrose-containing foods often show a higher nutrient (i.e. vitamin and mineral) density than traditional low-sugar food.

In System S, the Carbohydrate Boosters™ and recipes contain sucrose, but other nutrients as well. In other words, they are contributing healthy, useful things to your daily diet. Eating a variety of foods – some containing sucrose – is the best way to ensure that you get your fair share of good things. Excluding everything that contains sugar may not be healthy.

Many slimmers think that it is helpful to pick low-sugar items from the supermarket when they are trying to lose weight. Manufacturers were quick to recognise this trend and produce items with 'low-sugar' labels, mostly more expensive than the sugar-containing originals. A recent piece of research carried out at Reading University, England, has demonstrated that switching to low-sugar supermarket brands doesn't help slimmers. A group of women who chose sugar-reduced instead of regular foods when shopping did not lower their daily calorie intake at all. They just consumed the same number of calories as usual, making up the difference from other foods.

5. While You Are Eating a Mini Choc Bar, You Could Be Munching a Piece of Fruit

Yes, but why not enjoy both? There are times when it is easier or more appropriate to eat a choc bar or a couple of biscuits than it is to peel an orange or tuck into a juicy pear. If you are on the bus or in the office, it can be a messy, noisy business to crunch your way through an apple; nibbling a finger of fudge would be easier and far more enjoyable. On the other hand, if you are sitting at home watching TV after supper, eating an orange would be refreshing and you could easily pop to the bathroom during the commercial break to wash your sticky hands.

Social situations also make it difficult to be too particular about a choice of snack. For instance, if you are visiting friends, and they serve up biscuits with the coffee, it is very rude to insist on having a banana instead! With System S, you get plenty of opportunity to eat lots of fruit and sweets and chocs as well and you can eat them when it suits you and when they fit into your own lifestyle and eating pattern.

6. Eating Sugar Can Make You Become Diabetic

'Late onset' diabetes, the kind that hits people in their forties and onwards, is linked strongly with being overweight. However, it is not linked specifically with the over-consumption of sugar. Sufferers are now advised to follow a healthy, balanced diet which includes a variety of different foods. It is also now known that it's unnecessary to avoid sugar in food to achieve proper blood glucose control. Indeed, it is not advisable to do so. If you reduce your carbohydrate intake (including sugary foods) you are likely to eat more fat. This will increase your risk of heart disease. It is always advisable for anyone with a health problem such as diabetes to consult their doctor before following a specific weight-reducing diet. However, there is no reason why diabetics cannot follow System S, so long as they do so in consultation with their doctor or clinic. The British Diabetic Association now allows diabetics to have some sucrose-containing foods as part of their food intake.

7. *People Assume You Are Greedy if You Eat Sweets*

The truth is that most people are too busy thinking about themselves and their own problems to bother about what you are doing, unless you deliberately draw their attention to it. If someone who is very overweight tucks into a huge box of chocs with gusto in the middle of the day on a crowded train, he or she could be the object of a few knowing glances from fellow-passengers. However, if you are following the System S diet and include a sweet snack in your work lunch-box, no-one is going to think you are 'greedy' when you eat it, unless *you* give them that idea. **The important thing is to convince yourself that you are not greedy, or 'cheating' on your diet. Reading this book is the first step towards achieving a much more confident attitude towards food, and towards calling a halt to the self-mockery that so many overweight people use as a defence mechanism, often before anyone has actually been rude to them.**

Our System S 'guinea pig', Pat Aiton, became very secretive about her chocolate-eating habit, going so far as to hide her chocs from her own husband. Pat is now much more positive about herself and has changed her attitude. She eats her chocolate openly in front of her husband, John, and her friends.

Don't say: 'Look at me, I'm having a chocolate biscuit. Aren't I naughty?' You are asking for the response 'Yes, you are.'

Do say: 'This chocolate biscuit is scrumptious. Do you like this kind?' Your friend or colleague is then invited to talk about their own feelings and desires, instead of considering the question of whether or not you are greedy!

8. *Eating Sweet Foods Makes You Irritable and Cranky*

If you eat a balanced, varied diet, which includes some sweet foods, you should be able to maintain a healthy blood sugar balance. This means that you should *not* suffer from the sudden feelings of irritability or crankiness which may be caused by a sudden drop in blood sugar or (even more likely) the fact that you are being deprived of your favourite foods.

The old comparison between the human body and a motor car has been pretty well exhausted by diet book authors, but it still makes a lot of sense. You do need a regular intake of high-quality fuel to run smoothly. If you don't get it, you will slow down, seize up and you could break down completely. This is particularly true as far as our stressful lifestyle is concerned. We skip meals, then gulp down indigestible, high-fat snacks instead. No wonder we often feel irritable and depressed. The quickest way to feel more cheerful is to change your diet and eat sensibly and regularly. That means consuming an adequate amount of carbohydrate, plus other essential nutrients. Carbohydrate is particularly useful because it's the body's first choice of 'fuel' when energy is needed fast – and if we don't have enough stored in the 'pit stop' ready for use, the body then has to break down fat or protein . . . which takes longer. That's why it's so important for athletes to eat plenty of carbohydrate foods – see Chapter Six for more details of how System S can be tailored for sportsmen and women.

Lately, there has been a lot of interest in healthy diets which could be of value for women who suffer from pre-menstrual tension. Many women think they should cut out sweet foods altogether during the week before their period. In fact, this is not necessary. Eat regularly, drink plenty of water, avoid too much salt (which can aggravate uncomfortable bloating) and enjoy a few sweet Carbohydrate Boosters™.

9. If You Eat Sweets, Your Children Will Copy You and Get Fat

Children definitely do take the lead from their parents as far as diet is concerned. If parents eat too many fatty foods or too much confectionery, then their children are likely to do the same and suffer the same unpleasant health problems: weight gain, high blood pressure and even heart disease . . . but, suppose parents ban these foods? Then their children may consume them in secret anyway! So, what do you gain, except a child who is being secretive? If you bribe children with sweets, they will see them as something to be prized, sought after and used as tokens to 'swap' for good behaviour. This brings unnecessary pressure on parents and children and contributes to family dramas at supermarket checkouts and motorway cafés.

If you bring your children up to enjoy all kinds of dishes – fruit, vegetables, bread, cereals, fish, meat, sweets, chocolate – and make mealtimes an important and pleasant part of your family life, then they will have a good chance of developing a healthy, happy relationship with food. They will learn to eat normally, without guilt or hangups.

It is much better for a teenager to see his or her parents eating a whole variety of foods, including sucrose-containing foods, than to hear either of them moaning and groaning continuously about 'having to give up sweets' because of a diet. That is yet another good reason why System S is an excellent choice for anyone who wants to set a good example to teenage children.

10. Eating Sweets between Meals Ruins Your Appetite for Proper, Healthy Meals

Eating sweet foods plays an important part in helping to decrease your intake of fat. So, if your idea of a 'proper, healthy meal' is a plateful of greasy sausages, eggs, bacon and chips, then the warning about the dangers of eating between meals that every child is given at some time or other by well-meaning parents is perfectly valid. If you eat sufficient carbohydrate (perhaps a couple of the System S Carb Boosters™, for instance) and then sit down in front of a huge fry-up, you will probably leave a sausage or a few chips on your plate. For slimmers, particularly, to leave high-fat foods on the plate sounds like a good thing!

Eating sufficient carbohydrate, including sweet snacks between meals, helps cut fat cravings, but there is *no* evidence that it ruins your appetite for other things like fruit and vegetables. People living in the West are hardly ever truly 'hungry' (in the sense of being so hungry that some kind of food is vital for survival) but our appetites are triggered by all kinds of outside stimuli; advertisements, smells, even the sight of the hands on the clock registering 1pm or lunchtime. You are more likely to be led astray by sipping an alcoholic drink before dinner than by nibbling some sweets. A drink acts as an 'aperitif', stimulating your appetite, and also dulls the inhibiting mechanism of the brain which, subconsciously, tells you that you really don't need a large meal.

One additional note of interest. You may well be thinking that fat is often associated with sugar, for example in chocolate and cakes. Again, scientific research has come up with some interesting findings. As we have already seen, overweight and obese people have a definite preference for fatty food, which is why their diets are often high in fat. However, laboratory tests have found that it is the fatty foods associated with savoury and salty tastes (e.g. crisps, nuts or chips) which were preferred – *not* the fatty sweet foods like cakes and pastries. **While studies of groups of people have found that high-fat diets are linked with being overweight and obese, there is *no* link between sugar and excess weight.**

There are many good reasons for reducing the fat in your diet, but we prefer to follow a more positive message. *Increase* the carbohydrate, especially sugary foods, in your calorie-reduced diet, to suit your metabolism and your health. This is the successful formula for System S.

CHAPTER FOUR

'Test-Drive' the Diet

Once you start to follow System S, you will realise that it is very different from any other diet plan you may have tried before. As well as including sweet foods, it has a whole range of delicious meals (including dishes from Spain, Mexico and Thailand), snacks and even alcohol.

However, because the diet is so different, you may find that it takes a few weeks to get used to the plan. Suddenly, you will be eating foods that you may have deliberately tried to ignore on the supermarket shelves. Instead of dashing past the cakes, sweets and biscuits, you will be able to linger and make a proper choice from the foods available there. To say the least, it will be quite a shock to the system!

So, it is a good idea to 'test-drive' the diet for a few days before you start in earnest and even consider how much weight you want to lose. Choose a time when you can actually concentrate on yourself and your needs: when you get a week off from work and are spending the time at home, or when the children have gone back to school and you can look around the supermarket without lots of willing helpers to confuse you! This 'test-drive' will fit in well with a time when work is fairly routine . . . don't do it when you are up against deadlines all day long and feel under pressure. You could go off the rails and become disheartened.

If you are trying to lose weight with your partner, you could do your pre-diet trial over a long weekend. Don't accept invitations out to dinner but do invite people over if you wish. Don't even tell them that you are on a diet plan, until after they have enjoyed their meal!

On the following pages is a four-day plan to try. There are vegetarian options for non meat-eaters. Weigh yourself before you start and again, afterwards, if you like. If not, don't bother! Sounds like crazy advice for slimmers? This four-day 'test-drive' is more about finding out whether you enjoy the diet (you will, you will!) than whether you will lose much weight.

In any case, the System S is very different from conventional diets as far as weight-loss patterns are concerned. As any dedicated (and failed!) slimmer knows, the first week's weight loss is usually the most you'll ever lose in one week on that particular diet.

With System S the weight-loss pattern is more even; in other words, you'll lose less weight the first week than you will on 'normal' diets, but you will sustain that weight loss for longer, which means that, in the long run, you will actually lose *more* weight. You will also stay slim because your new eating pattern is so delicious and easy to stick to that you won't want to change it – ever!

This weight-loss pattern is different because, instead of cutting down on carbohydrate, the eating plan actually encourages slimmers to increase it. Here's why that makes a difference:

The body has two main ways in which it stores excess energy: as fat and as glycogen. Glycogen is always stored with water as an integral part of its molecular structure. The glycogen:water ratio is 1:4. When you reduce your energy intake (i.e. take in less calories than you burn off), the body will start mobilising its own energy stores. The first one it breaks down (because it is the easiest) is glycogen. When the glycogen molecules break down, water is released. Water doesn't have any energy (calories) but it is fairly heavy, so it contributes to your total weight loss. So, when people say, 'The first week on a diet, you lose most weight . . . but it's mainly water,' that is actually correct. So if you lose 2kg (4lb) in the first week of a conventional diet, you can be sure that only about 600g (1½lb) of that is actual fat.

When you follow a diet that contains carbohydrate in high amounts (like System S), the body is getting adequate carbohydrate which is easy to convert into glycogen, so it doesn't need to break down so much of its existing glycogen stores. However, as the *total* amount of energy (calories) is reduced, the body will break down a higher proportion of fat as well as some glycogen. Which means that, on your first week on System S, you will actually lose less water than on a conventional diet, and weight loss registered on the scales will be less than on a conventional diet. However, the weight loss is more likely to be fat than water. So, your true weight loss (i.e. *fat* loss) is exactly the same as on conventional diets, yet you have enjoyed all the foods that are banned on those diets, and you feel more satisfied.

With System S the weight loss, i.e. fat-loss pattern, is also much steadier than on other diets. The 'guinea pigs' who tried it found that they lost about 900g (2lb) the first week, then carried on losing weight steadily. There was very little 'jumping around' from week to week. This was because the diet sets a very steady eating pattern, which is simple to stick to and which gives plenty of carbohydrate, every single day.

So, how much will *you* lose? Once you start following the diet properly, you can expect a steady weight loss of at least 500g–1kg (1–2lb) a week, which means you could lose around a stone in two months. That is why you should not expect a big weight loss during your four-day 'test-drive'. However, you can be assured that the weight you do lose will be mostly fat, not water!

While you are following the four-day plan, you should *also* try out the Attitude Exercises listed on the following pages. These are important because they are designed to help you change your whole attitude to buying sweet foods and enjoying them. Some of them sound very easy – but for long-term, unsuccessful slimmers, they could be quite difficult. For instance, if you have trained yourself never to eat a sweet food, it could be quite difficult to change your habits. Don't panic. Just follow the tips given for each exercise and you'll find that they are a whole lot easier than you imagined.

Attitude Exercises
during Your Test-Drive

Day One

• Shop for two days' supply of your chosen Carb Boosters™ (see lists on pages 61–2). Go to a local supermarket and have a good look through the appropriate shelves for sweets, biscuits, cakes and frozen puddings.

• Buy at least one Carb Booster™ (such as a mini choc bar) from a pick 'n' mix counter or your local confectionery store. Chose somewhere you haven't been for a long time (maybe because you feared that you would be tempted to buy too many items or that people would recognise you as a 'failed' dieter).

Day Two

• Dare to eat a Carb Booster™ in a public place – on a bus, in a train, a restaurant or a shop. Eat it slowly and enjoy it. Do not glance around to check that no-one is looking at you. Just savour the moment. You deserve it.

• Eat another Carb Booster™ at home – in the most pleasurable surroundings you can imagine. Eat it in the bath, in front of the TV (not during a gripping programme, because you'll be concentrating on the drama on-screen instead of your own pleasure!) or lying on the sofa listening to a favourite CD.

Day Three

• Eat a Carb Booster™ in front of a work colleague or friend. Do not say, 'This is part of my diet plan, so it's OK to eat it.' Don't make any defensive remark. If they say, 'What's that you're eating? I thought you were on a diet,' respond by smiling enigmatically and making a noncommittal remark such as: 'I just fancied it – tastes lovely. Do you like them?'

• Try the same exercise. This time, eat the Carb Booster™ in front of a member of your family – husband, wife, partner or child. Make the same kind of positive response to any question they may ask about the item you are eating. Ask them if they would like one, too.

Day Four

• Invite someone to share your evening meal and serve up one of the delicious sweet puddings included in your diet menu. Again, be casual but positive about it. Do not apologise for serving up something 'naughty'. Do say that you hope they are enjoying it, as it is a new recipe which you are trying out for the first time. Maybe they would like a copy?

• The ultimate luxury – nibble a Carb Booster™ in bed. Make sure you choose something that's not too messy! As you enjoy your sweet snack, breathe deeply and imagine yourself looking slim and shapely at a party or other special occasion. Let yourself drift off to sleep, savouring both pleasures . . . the taste of the snack and the flattering picture of how you will look and feel after you have developed a new, happy relationship with food, and with yourself.

'Free' Vegetables:
Eat as Much as You Like

Before you start your four-day 'test-drive', check through the list of vegetables on page 56. You can eat them freely in all versions of System S, including the test-drive and the different plans in the next chapter.

There are several good reasons why it is important to fill up your plate with vegetables. First, the latest health recommendations emphasise the need to consume *at least* five portions of fruit and/or vegetables daily. Health problems like cancer, strokes and heart disease have been linked to poor consumption of both and there is definite evidence that eating adequate amounts gives you some protection against these modern-day killers.

Second, as well as being a good source of vitamins and minerals, vegetables contain fibre, which helps food to move through the body and keeps you feeling pleasantly full and satisfied. If you eat them raw, in salads, or lightly cooked (in stir-fries, for instance) they will retain their 'bite appeal' and fill you up at the same time. They also help make a meal look attractive and add bulk, so you never feel that you are sitting down to a pathetic portion of food, as you do on so many diet plans.

Third, and most important, there is really no point at all in limiting your intake of many vegetables because they contain so little energy (calories). For instance, lightly boiled or steamed courgettes or cabbage contain just 20 Cals for a 100g (4oz) portion and the same amount of carrots cooked the same way contain just 28 Cals. Even if you were a real glutton and ate a whole cabbage or 500g (1lb) of carrots at one sitting, the calorie total would be under 150 Cals. So, any diet that advocates weighing out small portions of either of these items, and of the others on our list, is not to be recommended.

Your 'Free' Vegetable List

Asparagus, Beans (Runner and French), Beansprouts, Broccoli, Brussels Sprouts, Cabbage, Carrots, Cauliflower, Celeriac, Celery, Chicory, Chinese Leaves, Chives, Courgettes, Cucumber, Curly Kale, Endive, Gherkins, Leeks, Lettuce, Mangetout (Snow Peas), Marrow, Mushrooms, Mustard and Cress, Okra, Peppers (red and green), Radishes, Shallots, Spinach, Spring Onions (Scallions), Squash, Swede, Tomatoes (Canned or Fresh), Turnips, Water Chestnuts, Watercress.

You can also have the following food items 'free' on the diet: garlic, herbs (e.g. parsley, dill, basil, tarragon), vinegar, lemon grass, Kaffir lime leaves (from large supermarkets and specialist oriental stores), lime and lemon juice, thin gravy, light soy sauce, Chinese Five Sauce, Chilli and Garlic Sauce, Worcestershire Sauce. All these good things will add taste-appeal to your salads and veggie dishes.

Great Ways to Serve Vegetables

Serve any of the vegetables above in huge, tasty salads, using either a light, fat-free vinaigrette dressing, or just a squeeze of lemon juice, vinegar, garlic, herbs and seasoning, or use any of the special System S dressing ideas on page 180. As well as including the more popular salad ingredients (lettuce, tomatoes, cucumber), experiment with other veggies, such as grated carrot, raw spinach, beansprouts, lightly cooked broccoli spears or sliced green beans.

You could lightly boil, stir-fry or steam the vegetables, either separately or in delicious combinations of two or more varieties. For instance, canned tomatoes taste wonderful lightly cooked with okra or courgettes, garlic and lemon juice; and celeriac combined with onion and carrot makes a wonderful purée which can accompany any meat or fish dish.

More Ideas for Vegetables:

1. Make shop-bought soups scrumptious: add freshly grated carrot, courgette, turnip or chopped mushrooms to a simple canned low-calorie soup to give it an individual flavour and make it more filling.

Dish up your own home-made soups. There is no need to add fat in cooking if you use a can of chopped tomatoes as a 'base', adding chopped onion, carrots and flavourings like garlic and herbs before topping up with softer vegetables like courgettes or grated cabbage and stock. Cook gently until all the vegetables are tender, and serve topped with a spoonful of natural low-fat yogurt on each portion. If you prefer a smoother soup, whizz it in a blender before serving.

2. Turn sandwiches into a whole meal: add salad vegetables to every sandwich to give it more flavour and extra vitamins. Try raw spinach and lemon juice with ham; asparagus tips, lettuce and lemon juice with smoked salmon or tuna; and chopped gherkins and peppers with low-fat soft cheese. When packing sandwiches to take to work, always include an airtight polythene box filled with a scrumptious salad to eat with them.

3. Make up a delicious thick tomato sauce for pasta and other dishes. Place the contents of 2 large cans of tomatoes with 2 tbsps of tomato paste in a thick-bottomed pan. Add 1 finely chopped shallot, 3 or 4 chopped, ripe, de-seeded, skinned fresh tomatoes, finely chopped garlic, lemon juice, a few basil leaves or mixed herbs and a little sugar to taste. Boil together for 15 minutes. The sauce freezes well, too.

4. Add plenty of vegetables to stews and casseroles. Root vegetables like swede, turnips and parsnips are particularly good because they absorb the delicious juices of the other casserole ingredients. They will 'bulk out' the meal, making more expensive ingredients go much further. They can also add colour and flavour, turning a simple everyday supper into something special.

5. Try serving vegetables chargrilled, Italian-style. There is no need to swamp vegetables in olive oil before roasting or grilling. Instead, wash and cut into chunks a selection of attractive vegetables such as red and green peppers, courgettes, tomatoes, onions, okra and squash. Place them in a shallow oven-proof dish, cover and cook in the microwave for a few minutes until they start to soften. Now, pop the dish under a low grill until the vegetables take colour. You can brush them with a little oil before grilling if you like, but they look and taste just as good without it.

6. Whiz up a stir-fry without even frying! You don't need a wok to cook a delicious, filling vegetable stir-fry. Just slice or chop a selection of vegetables. Start cooking by placing the contents of a small can of tomatoes into your wok or a deep non-stick frying pan. Add any onion and root vegetables first, then gradually add the softer vegetables. They will cook gently in their own juices. To add flavour and taste, add light soy sauce, lime or lemon juice, finely chopped garlic, seasoning and herbs.

7. Try braising vegetables in stock. This is a favourite continental cooking method and is very simple and economical if you are already using your oven to cook a roast or casserole. Simply place whole or sliced vegetables like chicory, leeks, parsnips or celery in a shallow casserole, add enough chicken or vegetable stock to come half-way up the vegetables, cover and cook in a moderate oven until tender, about 20–30 minutes.

8. Get stuffed! Try stuffing one vegetable with another. For instance, halved peppers taste heavenly stuffed with a mixture of tomatoes, courgettes and onion, then baked in the oven. Huge 'roast beef' tomatoes are scrumptious stuffed with finely chopped shallots and spinach. Marrow can be stuffed with just about anything, including chopped tomatoes, onion and garlic, water chestnuts, okra, carrots and spinach. Experiment . . . it's fun.

Carbohydrate:
Your Calming Influence

We are discovering what our grandparents and over half the world know – that carbohydrate cannot be beaten for its safe contribution to a healthy diet. We enjoy carbohydrate (and it is so nice to be told to eat the things you enjoy!). Carbohydrate has less energy, weight for weight, than fat, and scientific studies show that we quite happily replace fat in our diet when given the green light and are encouraged to eat our Carbs. So if you concentrate on enjoying Carbs, you can immediately, and with little effort, meet all the government targets for reducing fat. We are only just discovering the role that carbohydrate plays in appetite control and other areas (it may even affect brain hormones).

By following System S, you will:

- *Change* your attitude to carbohydrate: you *must* eat it and the allowances we suggest make sure that you get enough.
- *Change* your perception of vegetables: they are 'free', so eat lots.
- *Change* your perception of meals: concentrate on the carbohydrate and vegetables first (the meat, fish, cheese and eggs will look after themselves!).

To help, all the carbohydrate-rich foods in the diet plans that follow are shown in bold type.

★ Note: babies and young children don't need to concentrate on Carbs as much as the rest of us. If they ate only carbohydrate they'd have problems taking in enough food for growth. However, for adults trying to maintain, or even reduce, their weight, Carbs are great!

Carbohydrate Boosters™

On pages 61–2 are two lists of the Carbohydrate Boosters™ which will make this diet work for you. You must eat the number of Carb Boosters™ indicated at the beginning of your diet. In the test-drive, you are allowed two choices, but in other diets, this number may vary according to the amount of energy (calories) in your diet. Enjoy them at any time – between meals, after meals or just when you fancy something tasty.

Once the System S 'guinea pigs' had broken their own taboos about actually buying these sucrose-containing foods, they found it was best to stock up with a few days' supply at a time, and to plan out exactly when they would be eaten. Some of the diet testers found that a booster made a welcome snack half-way through the morning, others preferred to save at least one for late evening.

The Carbohydrate Boosters™ are divided into two lists: Low-fat Carbohydrate Boosters™ on page 61 and Medium-fat Carbohydrate Boosters™ on page 62.

Low-fat Carbohydrate Boosters™

All the Low-fat Carbohydrate Boosters™ have a high sucrose to calorie ratio – i.e. they contain a lot of sucrose (carbohydrate) for relatively few calories. They can be enjoyed at any time throughout the dieting week. Look at your diet plan to check how many you can eat each day.

Fruit-flavoured jelly (not the sugar-free kind)	About 1 bowl full	180g (6oz)
Crème Caramel	1 ramekin	100g (4oz)
Low-fat fruit yogurt	1 small carton	150g (5oz)
Skimmed sweetened condensed milk	1tbsp	25g (1oz)
Canned fruit in syrup	1 bowl full	150g (5oz)
Dried fruit	3 large (peaches) or 6 small pieces (apricots)	50g (2oz)
Raisins	1 heaped tbsp	25g (1oz)
Honey, jam or marmalade	1 heaped tbsp or 3 tsps	25g (1oz)
Golden syrup	1 level dsp	25g (1oz)
Boiled sweets, liquorice allsorts, fruit pastilles	5 sweets	25g (1oz)
Drinking chocolate powder/milkshake powder	1tbsp or 3tsps	25g (1oz)
Cola drink or other sweet fizzy drink	1 large glass	200ml (7floz)
Grape juice	1 large glass	200ml (7floz)
Chutney	1 large tbsp	50g (2oz)
Meringue nest	1	25g (1oz)
Fruit sorbet	1 scoop	50g (2oz)
Instant dessert made up with skimmed milk	5tbsps	150g (5oz)
Jelly Tots or Mini Jelly Babies	½ small packet	25g (1oz)
Marshmallows	5 large or 12–15 mini size	25g (1oz)

Medium-fat Carbohydrate Boosters™

You can enjoy these three or four times a week as part of your total Carbohydrate Booster™ allowance. Check with your diet plan to find out how many you may have each day.

Sweet cereals: e.g. Sugar Puffs, Smacks, Ricicles, Coco Pops, Crunchy Nut Cornflakes	6–7 tbsps	50g (2oz)
Arctic Roll	1 thick slice	150g (5oz)
Frozen mousse	1 small pot (about 1½tbsps)	100g (4oz)
Trifle	1½tbsps	100g (4oz)
Ice cream	2 scoops	100g (4oz)
Canned low-fat rice pudding	5tbsps	150g (5oz)
Low-fat custard (canned or in carton)	5tbsps	150g (5oz)
Home-made custard with skimmed milk and sugar	5tbsps	150g (5oz)
Jam sponge cake	wedge about 5cm (2in)	50g (2oz)
Jaffa cakes	4 cakes	40g (about 2oz)
Marzipan	1 piece about size of a large walnut	25g (1oz)
Popcorn (candied only)	1 large handful	25g (1oz)
Mars Bar, Curly Whirly or Snickers	1 'fun' size	
Chocolate buttons	20	25g (1oz)
Mini chocolate egg	4	25g (1oz)
Fancy, filled chocolates	4	25g (1oz)
Paynes Poppets	10	25g (1oz)
After Eight Mints	3	25g (1oz)

Wow! How about that for a list of delicious snacks? Don't forget, you *must eat* the number specified on your diet every single day if it is going to work properly. If you have consciously tried to exclude all these things from your normal diet, hoping that by doing so you will lose weight, then it could be difficult to remember which ones you actually enjoy. Try them!

For instance, you could start off by having a fruit yogurt after lunch. It probably won't taste very different from the sugar-free kind you have been used to (although it probably will have a fruitier taste because sugar tends to bring out the flavour). Then you could wean yourself on to a sugary soft drink before supper or a portion of cereal while you're watching TV. It's up to you.

The Four-Day System S Test-Drive

Plan of Action

1. Choose a time when you can think about yourself and can concentrate on your own needs – a long weekend, or when you have a few days' holiday at home, or during that precious lull when the children have gone back to school after the holidays. It could be helpful to test-drive the diet with your partner or a friend, so you can compare your experiences.

2. Read through the four-day plan and select the menu choices which you want to try. Pick your two daily Carb Boosters™ from the lists on pages 61–2 (don't forget that you can have different choices each day if you like).

3. Stock up with the food you need, plus plenty of the 'free' vegetables and extras from the list on page 56.

4. Each day, fill in the Food Diary on page 69, monitoring your own feelings by giving yourself points in the boxes where indicated.

5. Weigh yourself on the morning of Day One and again on the morning of Day Five.

6. At the end of the four days, check out the results of your food diary analysis on page 71.

Make Carbohydrate the Central Part of Your Meal

Traditionally we 'build' our meals around the protein- and fat-containing part of the menu and that item is always mentioned first. We talk about 'meat and potatoes' or 'cheese and biscuits', not 'potatoes and meat' or 'biscuits and cheese'.

However, with System S, it is vital to eat adequate carbohydrate – which means that foods like potatoes, bread, rice and your Carbohydrate Boosters™, are the most important items.

You can help yourself to slim more successfully by eating the carbohydrate-rich foods on your plate *before* the high-protein- and fat-containing items, whenever possible. So, if you are left with too much food on your plate, the 'leftovers' are more likely to be the protein- or fat-containing items than those containing most carbohydrate. For instance, if you sit down to a plateful of Chilli Con Carne (see page 176) accompanied by rice and salad, nibble some of the rice and salad before you plunge into the chilli dish. Or, if you are eating at a carvery, order a large 'free' salad as well and nibble some bread before you start eating the roast meat. **Try to change your thinking: carbs first, protein and fat last!**

As a reminder, those foods containing carbohydrate (including the ones rich in sucrose) are highlighted in bold type in each diet plan, including the test-drive.

Certain Things Apply Every Day

Daily Allowances

You may have 275ml (½pt) skimmed or semi-skimmed milk for your tea, coffee and cereals, unlimited water, mineral water and diet soft drinks.

Free Vegetables

Every day, include a good selection of 'free' vegetables – see page 56 for the full list. Add plenty of salad to bulk out sandwiches and serve a huge mixed salad or 'stir-fry' of vegetables with evening meals or at any time when you fancy a snack. Do not add fat.

For Men

Add 1 extra slice of bread or a medium roll or an extra Carb Booster™ or 1 apple, orange or pear and 1 extra glass dry wine or ½pt lager, beer or dry cider.

Alcoholic Drinks

Every day, you can have 1 glass dry wine or ½pt lager, beer or dry cider; or, save this up for a night out.

Day One

Carb Boosters™

Choose **two** items from the lists on pages 61–2. For example, how about a jaffa cake at tea-time?

Breakfast (choose one of the following)

- ½ small **melon**, 1 medium egg, poached, on 1 slice **toast**, grilled tomatoes, 1 carton (150g) **low-fat fruit yogurt**.
- 2tbsps (50g) **sweetened muesli**, with milk from allowance, plus 1 small **banana**, chopped.
- 4tbsps (25g) **sweetened cereal**, with milk from allowance, small glass (100ml) **fruit juice**.

Lunch (choose one of the following and don't forget the 'free' salad)

- Sandwich made with 2 slices **bread** and one of the following fillings and accompaniments: small can (100g) tuna in brine, drained and mixed with lemon juice, 1 **apple**; or 2 thin slices (50g) lean ham or cold chicken (no skin), 1 mug slimmer's soup , 1 **pear**.
- 2 slices **toast** topped with small can (150g) **baked beans**, grilled tomatoes, ½ small **melon**.

Supper (choose one of the following)

● Chilli Con Carne (recipe, page 176), 3tbsps (120g) plain, boiled **rice**, huge mixed salad from 'free' list, 1 scoop **fruit sorbet**.

● Birds Eye Cod Steak in **Wholemeal Crumb**, 2tbsps (100g) **mashed potato** (use milk from allowance for mashing), 2tbsps (60g) **peas**, 1 carton **low-fat fruit yogurt** or 1 bowl (180g) **fruit jelly**.

Day Two

Carb Boosters™

Choose **two** items from the lists on pages 61–2. For example, you might decide to have jelly with your Devon Custard tonight!

Breakfast (choose one)

● 1 rasher well-grilled back bacon, 2 slices **toast**, grilled tomatoes, mushrooms poached in water or a little stock, small glass (100ml) **fruit juice**.

● **Medium roll** with filling of 2tbsps (80g) cottage cheese and tomatoes, 1 large **banana**.

Lunch (choose one)

● Large (200g) **jacket potato** topped with ½ 375g can Buitoni Ratatouille (save the other half for tomorrow) and 1tbsp grated, reduced-fat Cheddar-type cheese, huge mixed salad from 'free' list, 1 **apple**.

● **Roll** or **bap** with one of these fillings and accompaniments: 2 thin slices (50g) any cold, lean meat with 2tbsps (90g) reduced-calorie coleslaw, 1 mug slimmer's soup, 1 **orange**; or 2tbsps (60g) low-fat soft cheese with chopped gherkins or cucumber, salad from 'free' list, 1 small **banana**, **apple** or **orange**.

Supper (choose one)

- **Raspberry and Kiwi Appetiser** (recipe, page 157), Piquant Fish Casserole (recipe, page 162), plenty of 'free' vegetables and salad, 2 scoops (100g) **fruit sorbet**.
- Any **pasta** – or **rice-based slimmers' ready-meal** such as Weight Watchers from Heinz or Findus Lean Cuisine with vegetables or salad with 1 pot (150g) Ambrosia **Low-Fat Rice Pudding** or **Devon Custard**.

Day Three

Carb Boosters™

Choose **two** items from the lists on pages 61–2. For example, Crunchy Nut Cornflakes before bedtime would be tasty!

Breakfast (choose one)

- 1 slice **toast** topped with grilled tomatoes, 2tbsps (80g) cottage cheese and Worcestershire Sauce to taste, 1 carton **low-fat fruit yogurt**.
- 2 **Weetabix biscuits**, with milk from allowance, 1 large **banana**, sliced.

Lunch (choose one)

- Small (75g) **pitta bread** stuffed with plenty of 'free' salad, plus one of these fillings and accompaniments: either ½ 375g can Buitoni Ratatouille, with lemon juice and 1tbsp grated, reduced-fat Cheddar-type cheese, a few **grapes**; or 185g can John West Oriental Crab or Shrimps with Crispy Vegetables, drained and mixed with lemon juice, 1 large **apple**.
- 1-egg omelette made in a non-stick pan with ½tsp olive oil for frying and filling of vegetables from 'free' list, 2 **crispbreads**, huge salad from 'free' list, 1 carton **low-fat fruit yogurt**.

Supper (choose one)

- Small (100g) chicken breast, skin removed and grilled with lemon juice, 'free' vegetables, 3tbsps (120g) plain, boiled **rice**, average portion (100g) any **stewed** or **soft fruit** with 2tsps **sugar**, or **canned in syrup**.
- Well-grilled beefburger, chickenburger or veggieburger in a **bun**, with small portion (100g) **oven chips**, grilled tomatoes, 'free' salad, 1 **apple**, **pear** or **orange**.

Day Four

Carb Boosters™

Choose **two** items from the lists on pages 61–2. For example, a slice of Arctic Roll after supper, perhaps?

Breakfast (choose one)

- Large bowl **fruit salad** made by chopping 1 large **banana**, 1 **apple**, 1 **pear** and topping with a few **grapes** and 1 carton **low-fat fruit yogurt**.
- 1 **Shredded Wheat** topped with 1 **chopped apple**, a few **raisins** and milk from allowance, 2 **crispbreads** with 2tsps **jam** or **marmalade**.

Lunch (choose one)

Crusty roll with one of these fillings and accompaniments: either 1tbsp (50g) Boursin Léger soft cheese or Kraft Light Philadelphia cheese, 'free' salad, 1 medium **banana**; or 1 pot Boots Shapers Reduced Calorie pâté, 'free' salad, 1 **apple**.

Supper (choose one)

- Turkey with Apricots and Ginger (recipe, page 159), 'free' salad and vegetables, 3tbsps (120g) plain, boiled **rice**, Boots Shapers **Strawberry Fruit Sundae** or Milk Chocolate Mousse.

• Small portion (150g) any **pasta** cooked 'al dente' (until just firm) and served with a sauce made from 'free' vegetables and medium portion (60g) prawns or cooked chicken (no skin), 1 carton **low-fat fruit yogurt**.

Four-Day Food Diary

Fill in your food and drink choices for the four days of the test-drive. Include meals, Carb Boosters™, alcohol and 'free' vegetables.

Give a maximum of 10 points for enjoyment and 10 points for satisfaction (i.e. how much it filled you up!). For instance, if your breakfast choice was delicious, and you felt very full afterwards, give it 10 points in each of the Enjoyment and Satisfaction columns. If it was only moderately enjoyable and didn't fill you up at all, then give it 5 for Enjoyment, 0 for Satisfaction. Add up the points in each column, add the daily totals together and then read the comments on pages 71–2.

Day One			
	Food and Drink	**Enjoyment**	**Satisfaction**
Breakfast			
Lunch			
Supper			
Carb Booster™ 1			
Carb Booster™ 2			
Total			

Day Two	Food and Drink	Enjoyment	Satisfaction
Breakfast			
Lunch			
Supper			
Carb Booster™ 1			
Carb Booster™ 2			
Total			

Day Three	Food and Drink	Enjoyment	Satisfaction
Breakfast			
Lunch			
Supper			
Carb Booster™ 1			
Carb Booster™ 2			
Total			

Day Four			
	Food and Drink	**Enjoyment**	**Satisfaction**
Breakfast			
Lunch			
Supper			
Carb Booster™ 1			
Carb Booster™ 2			
Total			

Grand Total			

Enjoyment

Between 200 and 150 points? Congratulations. The test-drive was a sweet success and you are well on the way to losing weight permanently. Your diet food choices appealed to your taste-buds and you can live with this kind of eating programme successfully. Don't forget to vary those Carb Boosters™.

Between 150 and 100 points? You are obviously not too happy with the food tastes yet. When you start a longer version of the diet (see Chapter Five), you will need to vary your choices and pick different Carb Boosters™. Try not to rush meals. Always eat your Carb Booster™ in a happy, relaxed environment . . . not when you are under stress.

Fewer than 100 points? Re-read your chart carefully and ask yourself the following questions. Are you so used to rushing meals that you never have time to enjoy them? Is there some kind of conflict at home which makes it difficult to relax at mealtimes? Did you cheat by cutting out foods? If the answers to any of these questions is 'yes', it could be a good idea to re-do your test-drive. Or you could fall into the category of 'inhibited' eater described on page 31. If so, you need to work through this problem.

Satisfaction

Between 200 and 150 points? Great – the diet is filling, so you know that you are not going to quit because you are hungry. You may even feel that you are too full. Remember that your 'free' vegetables are a movable feast – it's up to you when you eat them and how much you pile on your plate.

Between 150 and 100 points? Play around with your Carb Boosters™. If you have been eating both during the evening, switch one Carb Booster™ to the time when you are most hungry or tag a Carb Booster™ on to the meal which feels least satisfying. Are you eating enough 'free' vegetables?

Less than 100 points? Be honest – have you been missing breakfast or your Carbohydrate Boosters™ because you think you will lose weight quicker? Increase your intake of the high-fibre 'free' vegetables, such as cabbage, carrots or broccoli. Save your Carb Boosters™ for tummy-rumbling moments. Increase the amount of exercise you take and vary the times at which you take your meals, to stop yourself feeling hungry simply through habit.

What Did You Lose?

The main purpose of the test-drive is to establish whether the diet suits your food tastes and appetite and to make any adjustments you need. However, the bonus is that you should have lost some weight – around 500g–1.3kg (1–3lb). Remember that, unlike most other diets, this represents mainly fat loss, not water loss, so if your body tended to retain water, try the 'test-drive' for a further four days and see the difference. Now choose a plan from the next chapter. **The main thing is that you should *enjoy* this new way of eating.**

CHAPTER FIVE

Choose the Plan That's Right for You

If you enjoyed the System S test-drive in Chapter Four, you're ready to select one of the eating plans. How do you decide which one? First, find out how much weight you want to lose. Sorry, there are no handy charts in this book telling you just what you should weigh. That is because they can be misleading in the extreme, and often give slimmers a thoroughly daunting, idealised version of the 'perfect' weight. Quite honestly, there is no such thing. Everyone is different, and therefore there can be no rigid guidelines on the amount of weight that 'should' be lost by any individual, even if they are being treated in hospital for life-threatening obesity problems. Slimming clubs or clinics that force their clients to aim for unrealistic 'goal weights' are not to be recommended. Even losing 5kg (11lb) or so can make a difference to your health.

What is important is to decide for yourself what is a safe, sensible target to aim for. It may be that you remember a time not so long ago when you felt happy and healthy at a certain weight. Unless you have medical problems which prevent it, there is no reason why you should not get back into the kind of shape you were then. Perhaps you have always been overweight and know that you would feel a whole lot more agile and enthusiastic about your work and social life if you were several stones lighter? Now is the time to take control and shed weight gradually. Set some realistic targets: for example, 1 stone over a two-month period. Perhaps you are reasonably happy with your size and shape (even though you are not model-slim) but would like to lose just a few pounds because you feel 'middle-age spread' creeping up on you? Don't believe friends who tell you that it's impossible to stop the pounds piling on once you reach the magic age of forty. You can do it! However, it is important not to be unrealistic: for most people, simply shedding a stone or so helps change their lives for the better, with less risk of heart disease, high blood pressure and circulatory problems.

When you are deciding on the weight to aim for during your slimming campaign, remember to take into account your 'frame' – the skeletal structure of your body. Sorry but 'heavy bones' don't count. We all have bones, and they are not particularly heavy. What does count is your height, the width of your shoulders, your pelvic girdle, wrists and the size of your feet. You cannot hope to be the same weight as a friend who has narrow shoulders and tiny feet if you are broad-shouldered and wear size 12s!

Whatever the decision you make about how much weight to lose, it is your own – and you must feel comfortable with it.

To help you decide, the latest measuring device which is scientifically proven to be helpful in deciding just how much you would like to lose is the Waist Measurement Test (see page 28).

Next, read the following list of diet plans and see which one fits in best with your starting weight and lifestyle.

The diet plans are: Basic, Steady, Active Man's, Gourmet, Easy-Cook, Celebration and Maintenance. Plus, in Chapter Six, there are special plans for Vegetarians, Sport and Fitness Fans, and Teenagers.

Basic Plan

This is for women who want to lose between 3 and 20kg (7lb and 3st), and who lead a fairly sedentary life. If you are working in a sitting-down job and you are not more than 20kg (3st) above your desired weight, this plan will help you shed weight safely while you eat well. Even if you feel that you expend a lot of energy doing housework, and perhaps attend an exercise class once a week, you are still 'sedentary'. The average daily calorie count is about 1350 Cals, the carbohydrate count is 180g. It is not suitable for men, because even fairly lightweight males in sedentary jobs generally need more calories than non-active women.

Steady Plan

This is for women who want to shed more than 20kg (3st), or who lead very active lives. For instance, it is perfect for anyone who goes to an exercise class three or four times a week, or who takes part in active sports, but would still like to lose some weight. It is also suitable for men in sitting-down jobs, who take very little exercise. That includes those who would rather watch soccer on TV than actually play the game. It allows about 1500 Cals and 210g carbohydrate daily.

Although it may seem strange that a plan designed for women who want to lose this amount of weight allows more calories than one for those who only need to lose between 3 and 20kg (7lb and 3st), there are two very good reasons. First, if you weigh more than your slimmer colleague or friend, you need more calories to maintain that weight, therefore you can lose weight successfully by trimming away fewer calories than he or she can. Second, if you shed weight gradually you are more likely to keep it off.

Active Man's Plan

Men who are in fairly active jobs should follow this plan. It allows plenty of carbohydrate foods for extra energy and the portion sizes are very generous. It would also be suitable for women who are very active indeed or who have a lot of weight to lose (perhaps as much as 40 to 45kg/6 to 7st). However, once they have shed a few stones, it would be wise to switch to the Steady Plan. The daily calorie allowance on the Active Man's Plan is about 1750, with 230g carbohydrate.

Gourmet Plan

If you love a good night out at a restaurant and enjoy cooking interesting dishes, this is the plan for you. It allows about 1500 Cals and 210g carbohydrate daily, which means that it is suitable for most women and also for less active men. It's a good plan to choose if you want to slim down while you are on holiday or when you have a whole run of invitations and entertaining sessions in front of you. Those who love delicious desserts will be especially delighted with the Gourmet Plan.

Easy-Cook Plan

This is for those who prefer to spend as little time in the kitchen as possible. With the wealth of excellent ready-meals available in supermarkets and the popularity of microwave cookers, everyone can eat well without much effort. However, some people don't realise just how easy it is to rustle up 'instant' meals from fresh ingredients such as fish, eggs and vegetables. This plan shows you how. It allows about 1350 Cals and 200g carbohydrate for women with 20kg (3st) or less to lose and 1500 Cals and 220g carbohydrate for men.

Celebration Plan

This is a special, three-day plan for Christmas and other family celebrations. Unless you are very disciplined indeed, you are unlikely to *lose* weight during these festivities (although you might if you are very overweight, or you decided to cut back on the very generous booze allowance), but this plan will ensure that you don't put it on, either. You will feel in control of what you are eating and drinking, and yet you won't be a 'party pooper' either.

Christmas and other celebrations can present special problems for slimmers – or, they used to! System S is the only slimming regime that you can actually follow successfully during a two- or three-day family festival without feeling deprived of all the seasonal foods on offer, including the sweets and chocolates. During the 1996 trial of the diet, many of the 'guinea pigs' were so enthusiastic about the new way of eating that they asked for a special plan to be devised which took into account the fact that they might like to eat extra sweet foods and drink more alcohol at this time. This was duly done, and our diet testers reported that they were able to enjoy themselves without worrying about putting on weight. In fact, one or two actually lost a few pounds during the Christmas period.

Maintenance Plan

Once you have reached your 'happy' weight, this is the plan to follow. It allows you to introduce extra items into your diet, gradually, over a period of several weeks, so you can find the perfect calorie intake-expenditure balance to suit your own metabolism and lifestyle. It helps you learn how to vary your menus, enjoy eating and drinking and follow System S for the rest of your life. There is no set calorie or carbohydrate allowance, as this will vary with each individual, but make sure you put Carbs first.

Two factors to bear in mind, when choosing one of the diet plans, are your lifestyle and food tastes. If you are the kind of person who loves eating out at restaurants, then the Gourmet Plan is for you. Perhaps you are in a demanding job with very little time to prepare food, or live alone and don't enjoy spending a lot of time in the kitchen? In that case, you need the Easy-Cook Plan.

Maybe you are a very active man who needs more energy (calories) than most people in order to do your work. A diet which allows fewer than 1750 Cals could be unhealthy for you, and so the Active Man's Plan is the right one to choose.

Each plan is calculated to provide varied, enjoyable meals. The food and drink recommended are all available from supermarkets.

You may find that it is easiest to buy it all in one go during the weekly family 'shop', or in smaller amounts, according to your daily needs. It's up to you. Remember that the 'free' vegetables can be canned, frozen or fresh, but fresh is definitely tastiest! So, aim to choose your salads, other vegetables and fruits from your favourite greengrocer or market stall several times a week, rather than storing it in the fridge or larder all week. That way, you can be sure that you will get your fair share of the valuable vitamins and minerals fresh produce contains.

A note about sandwiches: because you are allowed unlimited 'free' salad vegetables, you really won't want butter or low-fat spread on your bread or rolls. Salad moistens and adds interesting texture, so you simply don't notice that there is no yellow fat on the bread. If you want to spread something over the bread to give it more 'bite', use a little low-fat salad dressing, mustard or Marmite before adding salad and your chosen filling. Remember – the bigger and more interesting the sandwich or roll, the more satisfied you will feel after eating it! Bread can be wholemeal, granary or white, whichever you prefer.

Shopping is a very emotive subject, and diet book authors love to give tips on how slimmers should go about it. 'Never shop on an empty stomach' is one favourite piece of advice. We recommend that System S slimmers try and shop as 'normally' as possible, that is at the same time and in the same supermarket or store as usual. If you decide to buy your week's supply of Carbohydrate Boosters™ all in one go, do so with a clear conscience. Don't try to hide your choc bars or biscuits under a pile of fruit or vegetables. If other shoppers give you knowing looks at the checkout, just ignore them. They may be hung up on the idea that all sweet foods are bad for you. Poor things, what an old-fashioned view!

Each of the diet plans provides adequate carbohydrate, protein, fat, fibre, vitamins and minerals for good health. They have been analysed by a qualified dietitian.

It is also important to vary your meal choices, so you get a good variety of different nutrients. If you stick to the same old menus every day (including your breakfast menu), you'll become bored and you could miss out on important nutrients.

You may swap the Light and Main Meals if you wish. For instance, it might be more convenient to eat a larger meal for Sunday lunch, then a lighter meal in the evening. Under no circumstances should you skip breakfast. If you really don't have time to sit down for breakfast, or oversleep, each of the plans includes several 'portable' breakfast meals which can be packed up to eat on the way to work, or when you get there.

* *IMPORTANT: if you are pregnant or have any health problem which necessitates a special kind of eating programme, suffer from a food allergy or allergies, or are diabetic, you should show your diet plan to your doctor or clinic before starting.*

Basic Plan

Daily Allowances

275ml (½pt) skimmed or semi-skimmed milk for your tea, coffee and cereals, unlimited water and mineral water. Drink diet soft drinks if you like, but water is best. No low-fat spreads unless specified.

Free Vegetables

Eat your fill from the list on page 56.

Carb Boosters™

Pick **two** items from the lists on pages 61–2 and eat them at any time, to suit your routine, either between meals or after a meal. Remember that Carb Booster™ cereal choices are **additional** to cereal at breakfast.

Alcoholic Drinks

Every day, you may have ½pt lager, beer or dry cider or 1 glass dry wine or 2 pub measures of spirits with low-calorie mixers only – or, save up your drinks allowance for a naughty night out! Instead of alcohol, you can have a medium glass (150ml) of fruit juice.

Breakfasts (choose one each day)

- ½ grapefruit, with ginger (if liked) and 1tsp **sugar**, 7tbsps (42g) **bran cereal**, with a little milk from allowance, 1 **banana**, sliced.
- 2 **Weetabix biscuits**, with milk from allowance, 1 **apple** or **pear**, sliced. 1 slice **toast** with 1tsp **jam**.
- 2 slices **toast** topped with grilled tomatoes, and small can (150g) **baked beans** with Worcestershire sauce to taste, small glass (100ml) **fruit juice**.
- Medium **bap** or **roll** with filling of 1tbsp (40g) **cottage cheese**, tomatoes, watercress, 1 carton **low-fat fruit yogurt**.
- Sandwich made with 2 slices **bread**, and filled with 'free' salad, and either small cube (12g) any hard cheese or small can (100g) tuna in brine, drained and mixed with lemon juice, 1 **apple**, **pear** or **orange**.
- 1 medium egg, boiled or poached, 2 slices **toast**, small glass (100ml) **fruit juice**.
- 4tbsps (25g) **sweetened cereal**, with milk from allowance, small glass (100ml) **fruit juice**, 1 slice **bread** with 1tsp **jam** or **marmalade**.

Light Meals (choose one each day)

- Sandwich made with 2 slices **bread** from a medium-sized loaf with one of these fillings, 'free' salad and accompaniments: either small cube (20g) hard cheese or 28g (1oz) low-fat soft cheese, 1 small **apple**, **pear** or 2 **satsumas**; or small can (100g) tuna in brine, drained, 1 small **banana**, 2 **jaffa cakes**; or 2 thin slices (50g) lean ham, cold chicken (no skin) or pork (no fat), 1 mug slimmer's soup, 1 **apple**, **orange** or **pear**; or 35g pot Princes, Shippams or Sutherlands fish or meat pâté or spread, handful of **grapes** or 2 **satsumas**, 2 **rich tea biscuits**.

• 1 well-grilled beefburger in a **roll**, mixed salad, 1 **apple**, **orange** or **pear**.

• 2 slices **toast**, 1 medium egg, poached, huge mixed salad, 1 **apple**, **orange** or **pear**.

• Medium (180g) **jacket potato** topped with either 2 thin slices (50g) chopped cooked chicken (no skin), mixed with 1tbsp reduced fat salad dressing, or 2tbsps (80g) **baked beans**, huge mixed salad.

• Large slice of **melon**, chicken drumstick (90g), skin removed, roasted, huge mixed salad or 'free' vegetables, 1 small **roll**, 1 **apple**, **orange** or **pear**.

• Medium portion (150g) any grilled or steamed white fish (no fat added, but plenty of finely chopped garlic, herbs and canned tomatoes, if liked), large (220g) **jacket potato**, huge portion 'free' vegetables and salad, a few **grapes**.

Main Meals (choose one each day)

• Medium portion (150g) any white fish, grilled, steamed or baked with lemon juice, 'free' herbs and vegetables and a little low-fat spread, large (220g) **jacket potato**, 1 **apple** or **orange**.

• **Oodles of Noodles Stir-Fry** (recipe, page 163), huge portion 'free' salad, 1 carton **low-fat fruit yogurt**, 1 small **banana**.

• **Spicy Vegetable Curry** (recipe, page 173), 3tbsps (120g) plain, boiled rice, 2tsps **sweet mango chutney**, huge portion 'free' salad, **fresh fruit salad** made with chopped **apple**, frozen **raspberries**, chunks of **melon** or **satsuma** segments.

• Lean beefburger (e.g. Birds Eye, 100% Beefburger), or Quorn quarterpounder, grilled, small portion (100g) **oven chips**, grilled tomatoes, 2tbsps (80g) **baked beans**, watercress, huge portion 'free' vegetables and salad, any **low-fat fruit yogurt** or Boots Shapers Dessert.

- ½ **grapefruit** or large slice **melon** with ginger, if liked,
1 medium portion (85g) any lean roast meat, thin gravy, 1 medium
(85g) **roast potato**, 2tbsps (20g) peas, large helping 'free'
vegetables, 1 **apple**, **pear** or **orange**.
- **Chilli Con Carne** (recipe, page 176), 3tbsps (120g) plain,
boiled **rice**, huge portion 'free' salad, medium portion (60g) frozen
raspberries topped with 1tbsp of natural yogurt.
- Any **rice-** or **pasta-based Weight Watchers from
Heinz**, or **Findus Lean Cuisine ready-meal**, huge portion
'free' vegetables and salad, 1 medium **banana**.
- Piquant Fish Casserole (recipe, page 162), large (220g) **jacket
potato**, huge portion 'free' vegetables and salad, 1 **apple**,
orange or **pear**.
- 3 thin slices (75g) any lean, roast meat, thin gravy, 1 medium (85g)
roast potato, 'free' vegetables, **baked apple** with 1tsp
sugar and a few **raisins** plus 1tbsp **low-fat fruit yogurt**.

Eating Out

Choose a meal from the menu that most closely resembles one
of the options above.

Steady Plan

Daily Allowances

275ml (½pt) skimmed or semi-skimmed milk for your tea, coffee and
cereals, unlimited water and mineral water. Drink diet soft drinks if
you like, but water is best. No low-fat spreads unless specified.

Free Vegetables

Choose liberally from the list on page 56, and pile them up on your
plate.

Carb Boosters™

Choose **two** each day from the lists on pages 61–2. Eat them between meals or at your 'danger' times – when you are most tempted to nibble. Remember that Carb Booster™ cereal choices are **additional** to cereal at breakfast.

Alcoholic Drinks

Every day, you may have ½pt lager, beer or dry cider, 1 glass dry wine or 2 pub measures of spirits with low-calorie mixers. Alternatively save up your booze allowance for one or two nights each week.

Breakfasts (choose one each day)

- ½ **grapefruit**, with ginger (if liked) and 1tsp **sugar**, 8–10 tbsps (50g) **sweetened cereal** with a little extra milk.
- 4tbsps (25g) **sweetened cereal**, with milk from allowance, 1 **apple** or **pear**, or 1 small **banana**, sliced, 1 slice **toast** with 1tsp **jam** or **marmalade**.
- 1 rasher well-grilled streaky bacon or 1tbsp (40g) cottage cheese or 1 medium egg, poached or boiled, 1 slice **toast**, 1 carton of **low-fat fruit yogurt**, 1 small glass (100ml) **fruit juice**.
- 2 slices **toast** topped with 5tbsps (120g) **baked beans**, grilled tomatoes, watercress, small glass (100ml) **fruit juice**.
- 1 mug slimmer's soup, any flavour, 1 slice **toast** spread with scraping of Marmite or 1tbsp (40g) cottage cheese, 1 medium **banana**, 1 carton **low-fat fruit yogurt**.
- Sandwich made with 2 slices **bread** or **toast**, or 1 medium **roll** with filling of 1 rasher well-grilled streaky bacon, grilled tomatoes, 1tsp tomato sauce, 1 **apple**, small glass (100ml) **fruit juice**.
- 1 medium egg, boiled or poached, 2 **crispbreads** with scraping of low-fat spread, 1 large **banana** or 1 **apple** and 1 **pear**, 1 carton **low-fat fruit yogurt**.

Light Meals (choose one each day)

- Sandwich made with 2 slices **bread** from a medium-sized loaf or a medium **roll** with 'free' salad, one of the following fillings and accompaniments: either 2 thin slices (50g) lean ham, beef, chicken (no skin), pork or other lean meat, or 1 well-grilled low-fat sausage, 1tsp **sweet pickle**, 1 mug slimmer's soup, 1 **apple**, **pear** or **orange**, 2 **jaffa cakes**; or small can (100g) tuna fish or salmon in brine, drained and mixed with lemon juice and black pepper, 1 medium **banana**, 2 **jaffa cakes**; or small cube (20g) Edam, Brie, Camembert, Feta, Red Leicester, St Paulin or low-fat cream cheese mixed with 1tsp **sweet pickle** or chopped gherkin (if liked), 1 carton **low-fat fruit yogurt**.

- Small can (210g) **ravioli** or **spaghetti** (not sugar-reduced) in tomato sauce, 1 slice **toast**, grilled tomatoes, 2 **satsumas** or 1 **apple**.

- Medium can (375g) **Buitoni Ratatouille** topped with 1tbsp (12g) grated Edam cheese, 2 slices **toast**, huge 'free' salad on the side, 1 medium **banana**.

- 1-egg omelette made in a non-stick pan with ½tsp olive oil, tomatoes, mushrooms, 1 slice **bread**, huge mixed 'free' salad and vegetables, 1 carton **low-fat fruit yogurt**, 1 **apple**, **orange** or **pear**.

- Chicken drumstick (90g), skin removed, grilled, huge portion 'free' vegetables and salad, 1 medium **roll** with 1tbsp (55g) low-fat soft cheese, 1 **orange**.

- **Spicy Vegetable Curry** (recipe, page 173), huge portion 'free' salad, 3tbsps (120g) plain, boiled **rice**, 1 **apple**, **pear** or **orange**.

- 1 beefburger in a **bun** (no onions), huge portion 'free' salad, 1 carton **low-fat fruit yogurt**.

Main Meals (choose one each day – and don't forget to add plenty of 'free' salad and vegetables)

- Chinese Lamb (recipe, page 169), 3tbsps (120g) plain, boiled **rice**, medium portion (60g) frozen **raspberries**.
- Medium portion (150g) any white fish, grilled with a little low-fat spread, black pepper and lemon juice, or cooked in a casserole with 'free' vegetables, large (220g) **jacket potato**, 100g (4oz) **peas**, 1 **apple**, **pear**, or **orange**.
- Birds Eye Quarterpounder or Dalepak Gammon Dalesteak, or similar large beefburger or lean gammon steak, small portion (100g) **oven chips**, grilled tomatoes, watercress, 1 slice of **pineapple**, grilled (optional), 1 scoop vanilla **ice cream**, 1tsp **strawberry** or **raspberry jam** diluted with water to make a sauce.
- Slice of **melon** with ginger (optional), 3 thin slices (75g) any lean cold roast meat (turkey, beef or pork), large (220g) **jacket potato**, small knob (12g) low-fat spread, lots of 'free' salad vegetables, 1 carton **low-fat fruit yogurt**.
- **Raspberry and Kiwi Appetiser** (recipe, page 157), 3 thin slices (75g) lean hot roast meat, thin gravy, medium (85g) **roast potato**, huge portion 'free' vegetables, 1 small **banana**, 1 small glass (100ml) **grape juice**.
- Mussels with Lime and Lemon Grass (recipe, page 172) with small slice **baguette** or any **rice-** or **pasta-based Weight Watchers from Heinz** or **Findus Lean Cuisine ready-meal**, 1 carton **low-fat fruit yogurt**.
- **Spaghettini** with Prawns and Garlic (recipe, page 167), huge salad from 'free' list, 1 **apple**, **pear**, or **orange**.

Eating Out

Choose a simple portion of meat or fish accompanied by a **jacket potato** or plain, boiled **rice** plus 'free' salad and vegetables. Choose **fruit** or a scoop of **fruit sorbet** for pudding.

Active Man's Plan

Daily Allowances

275ml (½pt) skimmed or semi-skimmed milk for your tea, coffee and cereals, unlimited water and mineral water. Drink diet soft drinks if you like, but water is best. No low-fat spreads unless specified.

Free Vegetables

Eat as much as you like from the list on page 56.

Carb Boosters™

Pick **four** from the lists on pages 61–2, and eat them at any time, to suit your routine, either between meals, after a meal, or included in a packed lunch. Remember that Carb Booster™ cereal choices are **additional** to cereal at breakfast.

Alcoholic Drinks

You may have 1pt beer, lager or dry cider each day, or 2 glasses dry wine or 2 pub measures of spirits with low-calorie mixers. Or save your alcohol allowance for weekends. If you are a non-drinker, you may choose 2 medium glasses (300ml) of fruit juice instead.

Breakfasts (choose one each day)

• **Saucy Beans on Toast** (recipe, page 145), 1 extra slice **toast**.

• 2 **Weetabix** or 2 **Shredded Wheat biscuits**, with milk from allowance, and 1 medium **banana**, sliced, 1 carton **low-fat fruit yogurt**.

• 1 medium egg, boiled or poached, 2 slices **toast**, 1 **apple**, small glass (100ml) **fruit juice**.

• Sandwich made with 2 slices **bread**, 1 rasher well-grilled crispy back bacon, watercress, tomatoes and mustard to taste, 1 **orange** or 2 **satsumas,** small glass (100ml) **fruit juice**.

- **Fruity Oats** (recipe, page 143), small glass (100ml) **fruit juice**, 1 medium **banana**.
- **Indian toast** (recipe, page 142), 3tbsps (120g) curried baked beans, 1 rasher well-grilled crispy lean bacon, grilled tomatoes.
- 7tbsps (45g) **sweetened cereal**, with milk from allowance, 2 slices **toast** with 2tsps **jam** or **marmalade**.

Light Meals (choose one each day)

Packed:

- Triple-decker sandwich made with 3 medium slices **bread**, spread with mild mustard or a little Marmite, lots of 'free' salad and two of the following fillings: either 2 thin slices (50g) cold cooked chicken (no skin), lean pork, ham or beef; or 1 portion (30g) Light Philadelphia Cheese Spread; or 2 Kraft Dairylea Cheese Triangles; or 2tbsps (80g) low-fat cottage cheese; or 1tbsp (10g) any hard cheese, grated; or 1 pot Shippams or Princes Sardine and Tomato Spread or Crab Pâté; or 1 rasher well-grilled streaky bacon, crumbled; or 50g (2oz) can of tuna, salmon or prawns in brine, drained and mixed with plenty of lemon juice and black pepper; or 3tsps **jam**, **honey** or **marmalade**; or 1 **apple**, sliced, with 1dsp **raisins** and plenty of lemon juice; or 2 level tsps peanut butter. Accompanied by 1 medium **banana** or 1 **apple** and 1 **pear**, 1 carton **low-fat fruit yogurt**.

(Don't forget that you can also add a **Carb Booster™** to your lunch-box.)

Eating Out:

- 2-egg omelette with lots of 'free' salad and 1 medium **roll** or piece of **baguette**, 1 **apple**.
- 75g (3oz) cold lean meat, or hot roast meat (e.g. chicken, beef or ham) with thin gravy, large portion 'free' vegetables and salad, 2 medium (100g) **boiled potatoes**, 2tbsps (60g) **peas**, 2 **satsumas** or 1 **orange**.

• Small portion **vegetarian lasagne** or **shepherd's pie** with huge 'free' salad.

Home-Cooked:

• Any of the **jacket potato** recipes on page 151, plus unlimited 'free' salad and vegetables and one of the following: 3tbsps (120g) **baked beans**, 1 carton **low-fat fruit yogurt**, 1 medium **roll**, 1 large **banana**.

• **Oodles of Noodles Stir-Fry** (recipe, page 163), huge portion 'free' salad, 1 slice **bread**, 1 **apple**, **orange** or **pear**, small glass (100ml) **fruit juice**.

• 2 slices **toast** topped with small can (150g) **baked beans** in tomato or barbecue sauce, or 1 medium egg, poached, or small can (100g) tuna or salmon in brine, drained, watercress, lettuce, grilled tomatoes, 1 large **banana**, 2 **jaffa cakes**.

Main Meals (choose one each day)

• 1 medium pork or lamb steak (120g), grilled or casseroled with 'free' vegetables and stock, 2tbsps (50g) **boiled** or **mashed potato** (use milk from allowance for mashing), 2tbsps (60g) **peas**, additional 'free' vegetables and salad, as much as you like, 1 medium **roll**.

• **Spaghettini** with Prawns and Garlic (recipe, page 167), huge 'free' salad, with Tomato and Basil Dressing (recipe, page 181), 1 carton **low-fat fruit yogurt**, 1 **apple**, **orange** or **pear**.

• Medium slice **melon** or **Raspberry and Kiwi Appetiser** (recipe, page 157), 4 thin slices (100g) any lean, cooked meat served hot (with thin gravy) or cold, with medium **roast** or **boiled potato** (85g), 2tbsps (60g) **sweetcorn** or **peas**, 'free' vegetables and salad, 1 large **baked apple**, stuffed with 1tbsp **raisins** and 1 tbsp **marmalade**.

• Birds Eye Cod Steak in **Harvest Crumb** or 2 Salmon **Fish Cakes** in **Wholemeal Crumb**, small portion (100g) **oven chips**, grilled tomatoes, huge 'free' salad, 1 medium **roll**, 1 **apple**, **pear** or small **banana**.

- 1 quarterpounder beefburger, well-grilled, small portion (100g) **oven chips** or medium (180g) **jacket potato**, grilled tomatoes, button mushrooms poached in a little water or stock, huge 'free' salad, 1 carton **low-fat fruit yogurt** or **fresh fruit salad** made from medium portion (50g) frozen **raspberries**, 1 sliced **apple** and 2 **satsumas**.
- Any Weight Watchers from Heinz or Findus Lean Cuisine **rice-** or **pasta-based ready-meal**, huge portion 'free' vegetables, 1 medium (150g) **jacket potato** or 3tbsps (120g) plain, boiled **rice**, 1 **apple**, **orange**, **pear** or small **banana**.
- 1 large (280g) grilled trout, 3 medium (150g) **boiled potatoes**, 2tbsps (60g) **peas**, huge portion 'free' vegetables and salad, 1 **apple**, **orange** or **pear**.
- **Chilli Con Carne** (recipe, page 176), 3tbsps (120g) plain, boiled **rice**, huge salad from 'free' list, 1 carton **low-fat fruit yogurt**.

Takeaways and Eating Out (have no more than one or two each week in place of your main meal only)

- Chinese: Beef in Oyster Sauce or Prawn Chop Suey with 6tbsps (240g) plain, boiled **rice**, 1 **apple**, **pear** or small **banana**.
- Indian: Chicken Tandoori or Tikka, huge mixed salad from 'free' list, cucumber raita, 6tbsps (240g) plain, boiled **rice**, 1tbsp **lime pickle** or **mango chutney**.
- Italian: **melon**, **pasta** with simple tomato or clam sauce (no cream), squid in red wine or mixed fish salad with 1 medium **roll** or 3tbsps (120g) plain, boiled **rice** and salad plus one scoop **fruit sorbet**.
- Carvery: **melon** or clear soup, lean meat – chicken (no skin), lamb, beef, pork (remove all visible fat and avoid the gravy), or simple grilled fish, 'free' vegetables, 1 large (220g) **jacket potato** or **fresh fruit salad**.

Gourmet Plan

If you love a good night out at a restaurant, and enjoy cooking interesting dishes, this is the plan for you. It allows about 1500 Cals daily, which means that it is suitable for most women and men in sitting-down jobs. It's a good plan to choose if you want to slim down while you are on holiday. Those who love delicious desserts will be especially delighted with the Gourmet Plan, and there is also a slightly more generous alcohol allowance.

Daily Allowances

275ml (½pt) skimmed or semi-skimmed milk for your tea, coffee and cereals, unlimited water and mineral water. Drink diet soft drinks if you like, but water is best. No low-fat spreads unless specified.

Free Vegetables

Eat as much as you like from the list on page 56, and experiment with delicious ways of preparing them.

Carb Boosters™

Pick **two** from the lists on page 61–2. If you like, you can add them to a meal. For instance, if you are eating out and fancy a couple of scoops of **ice cream** or **fruit sorbet** with your dessert, you can – so long as you count this as a Carb Booster™. When you are serving a meal at home, you may wish to hand round **After Eight Mints** with the coffee.

Alcoholic Drinks

Every day, you may have ½pt beer, lager or dry cider or 1 glass dry wine or champagne or 2 pub measures of spirits with low-calorie mixers only. You can also have a pub measure of dry sherry before your evening meal or a pub measure shot of brandy or whisky afterwards, topped up with water or low-calorie mixers only.

Breakfasts (choose one each day)

* Smoked Salmon Scramble (recipe, page 144), 2 **crispbreads** with 2tsps **marmalade**, small glass (100ml) **fruit juice**.

* ½ small **melon**, de-seeded, flesh chopped and mixed with 1 chopped **apple**, 1 carton **low-fat fruit yogurt**, 1 **satsuma** and replaced in **melon** half, 1 slice **toast** and 1tsp **jam**.

* 2 slices **toast** topped with grilled tomatoes, seasoned with fresh basil, black pepper and lemon juice to taste, 1 medium egg, poached, watercress, 1 small glass (100ml) **fruit juice**.

* **Lentil and Lime Kedgeree** (recipe, page 141), 1 **apple**, **orange** or **pear**.

* Gourmet bacon sandwich made with 2 slices **bread**, 'free' salad, 1 rasher well-grilled streaky bacon, crumbled, mustard and chopped herbs, small glass (100ml) **fruit juice**, 1 **apple**.

* **1 Shredded Wheat biscuit** topped with 1 **banana**, sliced, 1 carton **low-fat fruit yogurt**.

* ½ **grapefruit** with ginger (if liked), grilled until bubbly, 2 slices **toast** topped with 2tsps **raspberry jam** and 1tbsp **low-fat fruit yogurt**.

Light Meals (choose one each day)

* Super **sandwich** made with 2 slices **bread**, 'free' salad and one of the following fillings and accompaniments: either 2 slices (56g) smoked salmon, lime or lemon juice to taste and 2tsps low-fat cream cheese, 1 **apple** or **nectarine**; or 2 slices (50g) lean ham with 2tsps **dill pickle** or mild mustard, 1 small **banana**; or 1tbsp (50g) reduced-fat cheese, onion and chive spread (Weight Watchers from Heinz), sliced tomatoes and fresh basil, small bunch **grapes**.

* **Pitta bread treat** made from 1 small (75g) pitta, with one of the following fillings and accompaniments: either 2 slices (50g) sliced smoked chicken, Parma ham or Pastrami with 'free' salad, sliced gherkins or onions and mild mustard to taste, 1 large **pear**

or **orange**; or small can (100g) tuna or salmon in brine, drained and mixed with lemon or lime juice, 'free' salad, 1 medium **banana**; or small carton (100g) cottage cheese with chives or portion of Greek Tzatsiki (recipe, page 147), 'free' salad, 1 carton **low-fat fruit yogurt**.

• Medium **jacket potato** (180g) with one of the toppings on page 151, huge portion 'free' salad and vegetables, followed by 1 **apple**, **orange**, **pear** or small **banana**.

• Medium portion (200g) any white fish or small portion (100g) oily fish, grilled with lemon juice, served with huge portion 'free' salad and 1 medium **roll**, 1 **apple**, **pear** or **orange**.

• **Spaghettini** with Prawns and Garlic (recipe, page 167), with huge 'free' salad.

Eating Out
(for lunch, choose one of the following)

• French: Moules Marinières or **Crudités** with 1 small slice **baguette** followed by **Salade des Fruits** or **fresh fruit**, or 1 medium slice **baguette**, Camembert and green salad.

• Italian: Insalata di Mare (fish salad) with 1 medium **roll**, or **Spaghetti** with clams.

• English: Salmon or smoked salmon with salad and 2 slices **bread** and **fresh fruit** to follow, or 1 small, grilled steak or chop (remove fat) with huge portion 'free' vegetables, 1 medium **roll** and **fruit salad**.

• Pub: Cold meat or smoked salmon with salad, 1 medium **roll**, and **fruit salad** or **fresh fruit** to follow.

Main Meals (choose one each day)

All the following dishes are good enough for gourmet entertaining at home:

• Cantonese Beef (recipe, page 171), 3tbsps (120g) plain, boiled **rice**, 2 scoops vanilla **ice cream**.

• Thai Baked Trout (recipe, page 168), 2 small **boiled potatoes**

(100g), 'free' vegetables and salad, **Pineapple Slices** in Red
Wine (recipe, page 184) and 1 scoop **fruit sorbet**.
- Turkey with Apricots and Ginger (recipe, page 159) , 3tbsps
(120g) plain, boiled **rice**, 'free' vegetables and salad, 100g (4oz)
fresh fruit salad made with chopped **apple**, **pear**, **banana**,
lemon juice, **orange segments**, dash of Kirsch and mint sprig.
- Lemon Chicken (recipe, page 161), 'free' vegetables and salad,
Old-Fashioned Trifle (recipe, page 182) or **Pavlova** (recipe,
page 185).

Simple, easy-to-prepare, tasty meals

- 1 medium (150g) chicken breast or lean pork steak (75g) cooked
in the oven with tomatoes, herbs, finely chopped garlic and lemon
juice, 3tbsps (120g) plain, boiled **rice**, 'free' salad and vegetables,
1 carton **low-fat fruit yogurt** or 1 **baked apple** with 2tsps
clear **honey** poured over.
- 1 large (200g) mackerel or trout, stuffed with cooked chopped
spinach, grilled with lemon or lime juice, 3 small (150g) **boiled
potatoes**, 'free' vegetables and salad, small piece Camembert
or Brie cheese with 2 **crispbreads**, small portion (50g) **grapes**.
- Any **rice-** or **pasta-based gourmet ready-meal**
400 Cals or under (read the label), with huge portion 'free'
vegetables and salad, 1 carton **low-fat fruit yogurt**, 1 **apple**,
pear or small **banana** or small portion (50g) **grapes**.

Eating Out

This is where you must be careful not to go over the top – eat
out once or twice a week only, not every night! If you eat out at
lunch-time, make *that* your main meal. Good choices while you
are trying to lose weight are Thai and Japanese restaurants where
you can have simple, tasty fish and meat, with some plain, boiled
rice. Dangerous choices are Indian, Chinese and Italian restaurants where oil or ghee are used in cooking and which add lots
of fat and calories. It is safest to stick to the simplest dishes on the

menu, without creamy sauces. Start with plain, boiled rice, potato or pasta, then select from this list:

- Thai: Tom Yam Kung (Prawn Soup) or Thai-Style Salad or Nam Prik (crudités with shrimp sauce) followed by Tom Kha Kai (Chicken in Coconut Milk).
- Japanese: Fish Sushi, followed by Chicken Teriyaki or Japanese 'Roast' Beef with plain, boiled **rice**.
- Indian: Chicken or Lamb Tandoori or Tikka with salad and plain, boiled **rice**.
- Chinese: Stir-fried Beansprouts and Green Beans, Braised Chinese Leaves and Mushrooms, Sweet and Sour Cucumber, followed by Cantonese Braised Pork, or Crab with Ginger.
- Italian: Insalata di Mare (fish salad) or **Melon** with Parma Ham as a starter, followed by simple **pasta** with tomato or clam sauce (no cream).
- Carvery: **melon** followed by 2 slices lean meat with plenty of 'free' vegetables and 1 **jacket potato**.
- Steak House: **melon** or clear soup, followed by 1 medium rump steak, huge portion of 'free' vegetables and 1 **jacket potato**.

Easy-Cook Plan

This diet plan is for those who prefer to spend as little time in the kitchen as possible! With the wealth of excellent ready-meals available in supermarkets, and the popularity of microwave cookers, everyone can eat well without much effort. However, some people don't realise just how easy it is to rustle up 'instant' meals from fresh ingredients such as fish, eggs and vegetables. This plan, which allows about 1350 Cals for women, 1500 Cals for men, shows you how.

Daily Allowances

275ml (½pt) skimmed or semi-skimmed milk for your tea, coffee and cereals, unlimited water and mineral water. Drink diet soft drinks in moderation, but water is best. No low-fat spreads unless specified.

Free Vegetables

Eat as much as you like from the list on page 56.

For Men

1 slice **bread** or small **roll** and ½pt beer, lager or dry cider.

Carb Boosters™

Pick **two** from the lists on pages 61–2. Remember that Carb Booster™ cereal choices are **additional** to cereal at breakfast.

Alcoholic Drinks

½pt beer, lager or dry cider or 1 glass dry wine or 2 pub measures of spirits with low-calorie mixers.

Breakfasts (choose one each day)

- 2 portions **sugar-coated cereal** chosen from a 'Variety Pack', with milk from allowance, 1 **apple**, **pear** or small **banana**.
- 2 slices **toast** topped with grilled tomatoes and 1 well-grilled rasher back or streaky bacon, small glass (100ml) **fruit juice**.
- Sandwich made with 2 slices **bread**, spread with 1 triangle Kraft cheese, plus lettuce and tomatoes, 1 **apple**, **pear** or **orange**.
- 1 carton **low-fat fruit yogurt**, 2 **crispbreads** spread with a little Marmite or 1tsp of **jam** or **marmalade**, 1 small **banana**.
- **1 Kellogg's Nutri-Grain bar** or **Jordan's Frusli bar** with 1 **apple** and **pear** or 1 large **banana**.
- 1 medium egg, boiled or poached, 2 slices **toast** with Marmite, small glass (100ml) **fruit juice**.
- 1 **Weetabix** or **Shredded Wheat biscuit**, with milk from allowance, 1 medium **banana**, sliced, on top, 1 slice **toast** with 1tsp **jam** or **marmalade**.
- **Indian Toast** (recipe, page 142), 1 carton **low-fat fruit yogurt**.

Light Meals (choose one each day)

• Boots Shapers **sandwich** or **flatbread**, dessert and drink, to the total 'value' of 300 Cals. (There is a huge selection in this range. For example, you could have a Boots Shapers Prawn, Apple and Celery with Soft Cheese sandwich, plus a Lemon and Lime Yogurt and Wild Cherry Spring Water – for under 300 Cals). Add 1 **apple**, **orange** or **pear**.

• 1 large (200g) takeaway **jacket potato** with small portion (80g) baked bean filling and 'free' salad or vegetables.

• 1 can (400g) Campbell's Main Course Soup, any flavour, or 1 carton (568ml) **New Covent Garden Tuscan Bean Soup** or Smoked Haddock Chowder with a huge 'free' salad, 1 medium **roll** and 1 **apple**, **pear** or **orange**.

• 1 slice **toast** topped with 1 small (150g) can **baked beans** or **spaghetti**, tomatoes, watercress, 1 carton **low-fat fruit yogurt**.

• 1 medium **roll** or small (75g) **pitta bread** filled with one of the following fillings and 1tbsp of any low-calorie salad dressing (recipes on page 180); either small can (100g) tuna in brine, drained and mixed with 2tbsps (60g) sweetcorn; or 2 thin slices (50g) any lean meat; or 1 well-grilled (35g) low-fat sausage or bacon rasher; or 1 small pot tzatsiki; or 1 medium egg, hard-boiled; or 2tbsps (10g) grated cheese, any variety; served with 'free' salad and vegetables plus 1 **apple**, **orange**, **pear**, small **banana** or large slice of **melon** or 1 carton **low-fat fruit yogurt**.

• 4 **crispbreads** spread with 2tbsps (80g) low-fat cream cheese, 'free' salad and vegetables, 1 **low-fat fruit yogurt**, 1 **orange**.

Main Meals (choose one each day)

• Any **rice-** or **pasta-based Weight Watchers from Heinz** or **Findus Lean Cuisine ready-meal** or other ready-meal to the 'value' of 400 Cals (look at the label carefully), plus unlimited 'free' vegetables and salad.

- **Oodles of Noodles Stir-Fry** (recipe, page 163), huge mixed salad from 'free' list, medium portion (90g) **raspberries in syrup** with 1 carton **low-fat fruit yogurt** poured over and a handful of mini **marshmallows**.
- Turkey with Apricots and Ginger (recipe, page 159), 'free' vegetables, 3tbsps (120g) plain, cooked **rice**, 1 small **meringue nest** topped with small portion (60g) any **canned fruit in syrup**.
- 2 thin slices (50g) any lean, roast meat, thin gravy, 'free' vegetables, 2tbsps (100g) **mashed potato**, made with milk from allowance, 2 **crispbreads** and 1 Kraft cheese triangle or mini portion Brie, 1 carton **low-fat fruit yogurt** or small bunch (50g) **grapes**.
- 3 fish fingers or 1 portion white fish in **crumbs**, grilled, small portion (100g) **oven chips**, 'free' vegetables and salad, 2tbsps (100g) **mushy peas** or **baked beans**.
- Stir-Fried Tofu and Vegetables (recipe, page 170), 3tbsps (120g) plain, cooked **rice**, as much 'free' salad as you like, large helping **fruit jelly**, or 1 scoop **lemon sorbet** with medium portion (90g) **raspberries** or **strawberries**.

Celebration Plan

This is a special *three-day* plan for Christmas and other family celebrations. Let's face it, you are unlikely to *lose* weight during these festivities (although you might, if you are very overweight, or if you decide to cut back on the very generous booze allowance!), but this plan will ensure that you don't put it on, either. You will feel in control of what you are eating, and drinking, and yet you won't feel like a 'party pooper' either.

All you have to do is follow the *same* diet as you are following now, but with *two* additional items from this list each day:

- Small individual mince pie.
- 2tbsps (60g) double cream.
- **Small pork pie.**
- Medium **sausage roll**.
- 2 medium **roast potatoes** or **parsnips**.
- 2 mini chocolate swiss rolls.
- 6 squares of Turkish Delight.
- 20 **sugared almonds**.
- Medium grilled sausage.
- 6 **After Eight Mints**.
- 2 tbsps **bread sauce** and 2 tbsps **stuffing**.
- 2 glasses sparkling wine or champagne.
- 2 large sherries or glasses of vermouth.
- Small portion **Christmas pudding**.
- Small portion **fruit trifle**.
- 6 chocolate-covered nuts or roast nuts.

Maintenance Plan

Once you've reached your planned weight, this is the diet to follow. The calories are approximately 1500 for women, 1700 for men. It allows you to introduce extra items into your diet gradually, over a period of several weeks, so you can find the perfect calorie intake-expenditure balance to suit your own metabolism and lifestyle. Simply allow yourself a 2kg (5lb) 'ceiling' to account for bodily fluid changes. When you find that your weight remains under that ceiling permanently, you know that you are in business!

You can then plan your own food intake, week by week, going back on one of the other lower calorie diets if your weight creeps over that magic 2kg (5lb) top-up figure.

Here's how to use the plan. When you are happy with your weight loss, follow the basic diet below for two weeks. Weigh in at the end of this period. If you are still losing weight, add one of the 100-Cal extras on page 102 or another Carbohydrate Booster™. Follow the plan for another week and weigh in. If the pounds are still dropping off, add another 100-Cal extra or Carb Booster™ – and so on.

When you have established the perfect calorie level to maintain your weight, try to stick within that range. Don't be a slave to your scales! If the weight creeps up above that 2kg (5lb) 'ceiling', go back to your favourite version of System S.

Daily Allowances

275ml (½pt) skimmed or semi-skimmed milk for your tea, coffee and cereals, unlimited water and mineral water and diet soft drinks (but go easy). No low-fat spreads unless specified.

Free Vegetables

Choose them from the list on page 56.

For Men

Add 1 extra slice **bread** or small **roll** and ½pt beer, lager or dry cider.

Carb Boosters™

Choose them from the list on pages 61–2. Remember that Carb Booster™ cereal choices are **additional** to cereal at breakfast.

Alcoholic Drinks

½pt beer, lager or dry cider, or 1 glass dry wine or 1 pub measure of spirits with low-calorie mixers.

Breakfasts (choose one each day)

• 6-7tbsps (45g) any **sweetened cereal**, with milk from allowance, small glass (100ml) **fruit juice**, 1 **apple** or **pear**.

- 1 slice **toast** topped with 1 medium egg, poached, grilled tomatoes, mushrooms poached in water or stock, 1 small **banana**, 1 slice **toast** with 2tsps **jam** or **marmalade**.
- **1 Weetabix** or **Shredded Wheat biscuit**, with milk from allowance, 1 slice **toast** with 1 tsp of **jam** or **marmalade**, small glass (100ml) **fruit juice**.
- **Lentil and Lime Kedgeree** (recipe, page 141), small glass (100ml) **fruit juice**.
- **Indian Toast** (recipe, page 142), 1 carton **low-fat fruit yogurt**.
- **Fruity Oats** (recipe, page 143), 1 medium **banana**, 1 small glass (100ml) **fruit juice**.
- **Saucy Beans on Toast** (recipe, page 145), small glass (100ml) **fruit juice**.

Light Meals (choose one each day)

- 2 slices **bread** or 1 medium **roll** with one of the following fillings and accompaniments: either 2 thin slices (50g) lean ham, chicken (no skin), pork or beef or 1 well-grilled, low-fat sausage with 1tsp **sweet pickle**, 2 **jaffa cakes**; or small (100g) can tuna fish or salmon in brine, drained and mixed with lemon juice and black pepper, 1 medium **banana** and 2 **jaffa cakes**; or small piece (20g) Edam, Brie, Camembert, Feta, Red Leicester or St Paulin cheese or 1tbsp (25g) low-fat cream cheese with 1tsp **sweet pickle** or chopped gherkin, 1 carton **low-fat fruit yogurt**, 1 **apple**, **pear** or **orange**.
- Pasta Salad (recipe, page 149), 1 **apple**, **orange** or **pear**.
- Apple and Kipper Salad (recipe, page 146), 4 **crispbreads, 1 orange**.
- Large (220g) **jacket potato** with 3tbsps (120g) **baked beans** or one of the toppings on page 151.
- 1 well-grilled beefburger in a **roll**, 3tbsps (120g) **baked beans**, 'free' salad, 1 **apple**, **orange** or **pear**.

- Large slice of **melon**, chicken drumstick (90g), skin removed, grilled, 'free' salad and vegetables, 1 medium **roll** with 1 extra **Carb Booster™**.

Suppers (choose one each day)

- 2 lean pork or beef sausages, grilled, 2 medium **boiled potatoes**, 'free' vegetables and salad, 1 pot (150g) of **Ambrosia Low-Fat Rice Pudding** with a handful of **raisins**.
- 2 thin slices (50g) any lean, roast meat, thin gravy, 'free' vegetables, 1 medium (85g) **roast potato**, **Pavlova** (recipe, page 185).
- Mozzarella and Tomato Salad (recipe, page 164), medium portion (180g) any white fish, grilled, huge portion 'free' vegetables, small (100g) **jacket potato**, 1 **apple**, **pear** or **orange**.
- 'Free' vegetables, 1 lean pork escalope (75g), grilled, 1tbsp (50g) **mashed potato** made with milk from allowance, Figs with Parma Ham and **Sweet Yogurt** (recipe, page 188) or 1 medium **banana**, baked in the oven with lemon juice and grated nutmeg and served with 1 small carton **low-fat fruit yogurt**.
- Large plaice fillet (180g) or medium grilled mackerel or trout (150g), medium (180g) **jacket potato**, 'free' salad and vegetables, medium piece (40g) low-fat Cheddar-type cheese, 1 **crispbread**, 1 extra **Carb Booster™**.
- **Chilli Con Carne** (recipe, page 176), 3tbsps (120g) plain, boiled **rice**, 'free' salad, 1 **apple**, **orange** or **pear**.
- 1 well-grilled beefburger, small portion (130g) **oven chips**, grilled tomatoes, small can (150g) **baked beans**, 'free' salad and vegetables, 1 carton **low-fat fruit yogurt**.
- **Spaghettini** with Prawns and Garlic (recipe, page 167) or medium portion (230g) any **pasta** with 3tbsps (100g) Bolognese sauce made from lean minced lamb or beef, canned tomatoes, herbs and finely chopped garlic and 2tsps grated Parmesan cheese, 'free' salad.

100-Cal extras

Each of these items will provide an extra 100 Cals.

- 1 slice **bread** or 1 small **roll**.
- 2 thin slices lean meat.
- Medium portion (150g) white fish or shellfish, poached or grilled, with no fat added.
- 2 heaped tbsps (80g) **mushy peas** or 3tbsps (90g) **butter beans**.
- 1 chocolate digestive **biscuit**.
- 2 small new **potatoes** or 2tbsps (100g) **mashed potato** (made with milk from allowance).
- Small portion (130g) **oven chips**.
- ½pt beer, lager or dry cider or 1 glass dry wine or 2 pub measures of spirits with low-calorie mixers.
- 1 low-fat **Carb Booster**™.

CHAPTER SIX

Special Plans
for Special People

Are you a slimmer who happens to be vegetarian? Or someone who wants to shape up for sport? Or a growing teenager who is worried about 'puppy fat'? If you are one of these 'special' people with particular dietary needs, then System S can work for you. Because it is rich in carbohydrate, and low in fat, the diet is very healthy indeed. It also provides the vitamins and minerals we all need to stay in top form, and is so versatile that it can be adapted to suit all incomes, ages, and tastes.

Vegetarians

Vegetarians can easily follow the diet. All you have to do is try the special version on page 105. You will find that the Recipe Section (from page 139 onwards) includes imaginative ideas for meat-free breakfasts, lunches, suppers and snacks which you can also use if you want to plan your own version of System S (the recipes are all calorie-counted to help you devise your own menus). The Carbohydrate Boosters™, which are such an important part of the diet, are all meat-free, so these can be incorporated into your daily food plan with no extra bother. Remember that it is very important for vegetarians to eat a varied diet which includes fresh fruit, green vegetables, peas and beans, dairy produce, nuts and seeds. There is certainly no need to go short of protein – animal products are, gram for gram, only a very slightly better source of protein than nuts or seeds and no better than things like soya beans. Don't forget that carbohydrate-rich foods like bread, cereals, rice and pasta also contain some protein and these foods are eaten in quite large quantities on System S. Once inside your body, proteins, whether from meat or plants, are broken down into their component parts – the source is not important, so long as there is a regular supply!

If you are someone who has recently become a vegetarian (or who fancies changing their meat-eating habits for a few weeks or months), the diet is especially valuable. It helps teach you how to plan varied meals with the minimum of fuss and provides lots of ideas. Some 'veggies' do experience weight-gain when they first give up meat-eating, but this is usually because they simply substitute high-fat foods for the meat or fish that used to be the central item on the menu. They fill the empty space on their plate (and in their tummy!) with more chips, an extra helping of bread and butter, or have a second portion of pud with additional cream or ice cream afterwards. This happens very easily if you are someone who has decided to 'give up' animal products (i.e. deprive yourself of a whole range of foods), instead of being positive and enjoying the multitude of exciting food choices that are now available to vegetarians. Instead of planning your meal around an empty space, make your vegetarian main dish the focus of your meal and investigate the exciting cuisines enjoyed in countries where meat is not always on the menu. Try cooking with Tofu and Quorn – both absorb flavours from other foods and add bulk and texture to your cooking. Try the Spicy Vegetable Curry on page 174, the Stir-Fried Tofu and Vegetables on page 170 or, if you are really hungry, go for Boston Baked Beans on page 160.

One of the best developments for vegetarian gourmets in recent years is that now virtually every restaurant can provide at least one imaginative vegetarian main course dish. Most good restaurants take a pride in producing tasty meat-free and fish-free casseroles, pasta and rice dishes. Best are the ethnic restaurants such as Italian, Thai, Indian and Chinese. Professor Anne de Looy, co-author of this book, is a vegetarian and she rarely has to complain about the lack of choice. She has some tips for those who are following the diet: 'Vegetarian System S dieters can easily eat out while they slim,' she says. 'They can choose from first courses like vegetable soups, melon, pasta dishes, pick a whole range of main courses and, unlike most diets, they are also encouraged to have a sweet pudding. There is no need to check whether the fresh fruit salad contains sugar, or the fruit sorbet is sweet – if they *do* contain sucrose, so much the better!'

Vegetarian Plan

This plan is suitable for all vegetarians, but not for vegans (a vegan eats no animal fat at all – no eggs, milk or animal-based produce). It is also a good plan to follow if you are a non-vegetarian who fancies a change! The calorie count is 1500 Cals and 220g carbohydrate daily. Men who have 'heavy duty' jobs or who take regular exercise should increase their Carbohydrate Boosters™ and eat extra bread. (See the Sports Fans section on page 108, for guidelines.)

Daily Allowances

275ml (½pt) skimmed or semi-skimmed milk for your tea, coffee and cereals, unlimited water and mineral water. Drink diet soft drinks if you like, but water is best. No low-fat spreads unless specified.

Free Vegetables

The list on page 56 is obviously very useful for you, and do try all the tips and ideas given on how to use them.

Carb Boosters™

Choose **two** (or more if you are very active) from the lists on pages 61–2. Remember that Carb Booster™ cereal choices are **additional** to cereal at breakfast.

Alcoholic Drinks

You can have ½pt beer, lager or dry cider or 2 pub measures of spirits with low-calorie mixers each day, or save them up for a couple of nights out. Non-drinkers can have 2 medium glasses (300ml) of fruit juice.

Breakfasts (choose one each day)

- 1 **Weetabix biscuit**, with milk from allowance, 1 slice **toast**, 1 large **banana**.
- 2 slices **toast** topped with 1 medium egg, poached, watercress, grilled tomatoes, mushrooms poached in a little water or stock, 1 **apple** or **orange**.
- 1 carton **low-fat fruit yogurt**, 2 **crispbreads** spread with 1tbsp (40g) cottage cheese and sliced tomatoes, 1 **apple** or **pear**.
- **Fruit salad** made with medium portion (50g) frozen **raspberries**,1 sliced **nectarine** or **peach**, 1 chopped **apple**, a few **grapes** and topped with 1 heaped tbsp (50g) **low-fat fruit yogurt** and 2tbsps (30g) of **sweetened muesli**.
- 7tbsps (45g) any **sweetened cereal**, with milk from allowance, 1 **apple**, **orange** or **pear**.
- 1 slice **toast** topped with 3tbsps (120g) **baked beans**, grilled tomatoes, watercress, small glass (100ml) **fruit juice**.

Light Meals (choose one each day)

- Sandwich made with 2 slices **bread** or 1 crusty **roll** with 'free' salad and one of the following fillings and accompaniments: either 1 small **banana**, mashed with lemon juice to taste, 1tbsp (25g) **low-fat fruit yogurt**, a few **grapes**; or pot (75g) Boots Shapers Mushroom and Herb or Spinach and Lentil pâté, 1 **apple**, **orange** or small **banana**; or 2tbsps (30g) **Heinz Sandwich Spread**, 1 **satsuma**, medium piece (40g) reduced-fat Cheddar cheese; or 1 jar (50g) Shippams Chilli Bean spread, 2 **plums** or 1 **pear** and 2 **jaffa cakes**.

- Large (220g) **jacket potato** with any suitable topping from the list on page 151, plus huge portion 'free' salad, 1 **apple**, **orange** or small **banana**.
- **Pasta Salad** (recipe, page 149), 'free' salad.
- 2 slices **toast** or 1 medium **roll**, with one of the following toppings or fillings, a huge 'free' salad and accompaniment: either Quorn Southern Style Burger or other vegetable burger or 2 small **vegetarian sausages**, watercress, tomatoes, 1 **choc ice**; or 2tbsps (50g) Light Philadelphia Soft Cheese or other low-fat cheese, cucumber, tomatoes, 6 dried **apricot halves**.
- 3tbsps (150g) Sainsbury's **Ratatouille Provençale**, or other ratatouille mixed with lemon juice and 1tsp grated Parmesan cheese, 1 **pear** and a handful of mini **marshmallows**.
- Greek Tzatsiki (recipe, page 147), 1 **apple**, **pear** or **orange** and 2 **jaffa cakes**.

Main Meals (choose one each day)

- **Boston Baked Beans** (recipe, page 160), 3tbsps (120g) plain, boiled **rice**, huge portion 'free' vegetables and salad, 1 **baked apple** with 1tsp clear **honey**.
- Stir-Fried Tofu and Vegetables (recipe, page 170), 3tbsps (120g) plain, boiled **rice**, huge portion 'free' salad, **Pineapple Slices** in Red Wine (recipe, page 184).
- Cauliflower Cheese, made from as much cauliflower as you like with a sauce made from 2tbsps (20g) grated Edam cheese, 25g low-fat spread, 1 level tbsp (20g) **flour** and 275ml (½pt) skimmed milk. Serve with grilled tomatoes, 2tbsps (60g) **peas**, huge 'free' salad, 1 **apple**, **orange** or **pear**.
- 1 can (400g) **Crosse and Blackwell Healthy Balance Vegetable Ravioli**, grilled tomatoes, huge 'free' salad and vegetables, 1 medium **roll**, 1 scoop **fruit sorbet**.
- Large slice of **melon** with ginger, if liked, **Spinach Lasagne** (recipe, page 165), huge 'free' salad,

- McCain **Deep Crust Cheese, Vegetable and Tomato Pizza** or **Spicy Vegetable Curry** (recipe, page 173), 3tbsps (120g) plain, boiled rice, huge 'free' salad, 1 **apple**, **orange** or small **banana**.
- Any **rice-** or **pasta-based vegetarian ready-meal** that has 400 Cals or under with huge portion 'free' vegetables and salad.

Eating Out

Choose low-fat foods, such as melon or salads, but beware of vegetarian 'specials' which are often made with lots of cream, cheese and oil!

Sport and Fitness Fans

Sports enthusiasts, or those who have recently started following an exercise or training programme will find that System S is the best ever plan for good sports nutrition. It helps ensure that you get your fair share of all the nutrients you require, especially carbohydrates, which are the primary energy source when you are exercising. As was explained in the first three chapters, with System S, carbohydrate supplies are boosted to a level which is difficult to obtain simply by consuming traditional 'carb-loading' foods like pasta, rice and potatoes. By incorporating the special Carbohydrate Boosters™ into your healthy diet plan, alongside the complex carbohydrate foods above, you will be able to ensure that your carbs are 'topped up' regularly.

By now, most sports fans (even the armchair variety!) will know that it is a good idea to cut back on fat. If you are exercising regularly, your calorie needs will be more than if you are a couch potato, even if you are trying to lose some weight as well. A common mistake that even top athletes can make is to reduce their fat intake without replacing those calories with adequate carbohydrate to make up the daily total required.

There are three levels of exercise you may be already taking or hope to take: 'low-level' exercise like a swim at the local pool, a brisk walk, an aerobics class or a round of golf once or twice a week; 'regular commitment' like a jog each morning, a few lengths of the pool at lunchtime or a work-out at the gym three or four times a week; and 'training' involving joining a club with a programme of regular training leading to competitions, games or matches.

At each level, the proportion of fat to muscle is important. Generally, unless you are a long-distance Channel swimmer, you will exercise more easily, get less out of breath and be more agile if you carry less fat. You may be anxious that if you try to reduce your weight you will lose muscle or won't have sufficient energy to carry on with your exercise routine. Don't worry: if you stick to the Sport and Fitness Plan (see page 112) you will lose body fat – and have plenty of energy as well.

All exercise increases your calorie needs. Obviously, the longer you do the exercise, and the more vigorous it is, the more energy you will need. (Incidentally, when you do exercise you release a body hormone which makes you feel really good – so exercise also improves your whole outlook on life.) The body burns a mixture of fat and carbohydrate to provide the energy for the exercise, but it doesn't keep a large store of carbohydrate (although there may be plenty of fat!). So, the amount of exercise you can do is limited by how fit you are and your store of carbohydrate. If you are on a traditional weight-loss diet, the chances are that you will have cut out a lot of carbohydrate foods and therefore you will reduce even more the amount of exercise you can manage. You will know when you have run out of carbohydrate stores because you will feel really tired, your legs or arms get that heavy feeling and you can't carry on. That is rather self-defeating when you are trying to increase the amount of exercise you take to improve your form.

For instance, if you are a woman who is 13kg (2st) overweight and you enjoy a 20-minute work-out in the gym three or four times a week or go swimming every day, you will need more calories than your friend who weighs the same as you but doesn't exercise. He or she may well be following a diet which allows around 1250 Cals daily but *you* should not cut your daily calorie intake below 1500 Cals – even if you want to slim and are cutting back on fat. By nibbling a couple of Carbohydrate Boosters™ during the day, you will effectively top up your calories and your carbohydrate while helping to reduce your craving for fat. You can also use your 'CB™', combined with fruit, as a 'pre-exercise' or 'post-exercise' snack. Sally Ann Voak, co-author of this book, goes for an hour-long work-out and swim two or three times a week. Before leaving for her fitness club, she has a small carton of low-fat fruit yogurt (a 'CB™') and an apple. After her exercise session, she drinks a large glass of mineral water, eats a medium banana (to replace fluid and potassium) and nibbles another 'CB™', this time 3 toffees or boiled sweets, while driving back to her office.

As you can see, for the person who takes 'low-level' exercise, there is no need to increase CBs™. This type of exercise will not make extra demands on their carbohydrate stores. However, the person who makes a 'regular commitment' to exercise will probably need to increase their CBs™ by one or two each day. Don't take them just before you exercise because the body cannot get them into the system fast enough to be useful. Take the CBs™ after exercise or, even better, spread throughout the day. If you find that the weight is not coming off as rapidly as you'd like, then reduce the CBs™ one at a time.

If you are a person who 'trains', then you really need to seek special help with your diet. How many CBs™ you will need depends on your exercise schedule, but an extra four or five daily may be necessary. The very best way to test how well you are doing is to ask yourself this simple question: can you do as much training as before you started the diet, and is it getting easier? If the answer is 'yes' then it's likely that you are getting sufficient CBs™.

Of course, some top athletes and sportsmen and women need a lot more calories than the rest of us. A 1.9m (6ft 2in) professional football player who trains every day and plays a tough match on Saturdays, needs as much as 3500 Cals daily. If he simply relies on munching his way through piles of pasta with low-fat sauces to provide these extra calories he will find that he cannot manage to eat all the pasta, and when his tummy starts rumbling he could be tempted to 'top up' with a high-fat snack food. By incorporating four, five or even six Carbohydrate Boosters™ in his daily diet, as snacks or part of snacks (perhaps eaten with fruit or a sandwich), he will get the extra carbohydrate and calories he needs without having to resort to taking in more fat than is healthy.

When you get to this level of additional CBs™ you should introduce some additional bread to your diet rather than go on increasing the number of CBs™. At this level, you really need to experiment with what suits your lifestyle best. Just like the person taking 'regular' exercise, you must spread your CBs™ throughout the day, and not just before you train. Also, remember it takes about 24 hours for the carbohydrate (glycogen) stores to build up, so don't expect to do a heavy training session one day and then be able to do the same the next. You need to give your body time to build up its stores. Vary your calorie intake when you train seasonally. For example, if football is your sport, the summer is the time to reduce your calories and your CBs™, otherwise you will find yourself in an unhealthy 'yo-yo' weight gain and loss pattern.

Some people who train or exercise for periods of longer than 45 minutes at any one time will find that taking small amounts of carbohydrate while exercising helps to prolong their performance. A CB™ such as a cola drink or other fluid is probably the best choice as it is rapidly absorbed and tops up fluid at the same time. Remember that even though it will be used up quickly, it still needs to be part of your diet, not additional to it.

Whatever your exercise level, remember that the body sweats and also loses water in the air we breathe out (on a cold day, you can actually see this water being exhaled). It needs to be replaced (by water, not alcohol!). Even swimmers sweat into the water and need to take in fluid after their swim. Dehydration can cause poor exercise performance, and can also seriously affect your concentration, leading to accidents. Be careful.

As we said in Chapter Two, taking regular exercise is a great idea for slimmers. It will help you to stick to your diet and make the results more lasting. You will also tone up your wobbles while you slim. If you are very overweight, it is a good idea to start off simply by walking more: wear comfortable clothes and shoes, leave heavy shopping bags at home, and walk for 20 minutes or so each day. Once you become confident (and have lost a little weight), the next step is to do a gentle work-out, with an exercise video at home or at an aquarobics session in your local pool. These are fun and attract people of all shapes and sizes so you won't feel embarrassed even if you are still overweight. If you join a gym or sports club, make sure that the staff are friendly and well-trained.

Sport and Fitness Plan

This diet plan is for those on a 'low-level' or 'regular commitment' kind of exercise programme, who also want to lose some weight. It allows 1500–1750 Cals daily and 220–250g carbohydrate daily. It is not suitable for anyone on a 'training' kind of exercise programme, who should consult their club nutritionist about a suitable diet programme, taking into account the tips given in this chapter.

Daily Allowances

275ml (½pt) skimmed or semi-skimmed milk for your tea, coffee and cereals, unlimited water and mineral water. Drink diet soft drinks if you like, but water is best. No low-fat spreads are to be used unless specified.

Free Vegetables

Choose them from the list on page 56.

Carb Boosters™

Choose **two** to **four** each day from the lists on pages 61–2. If your exercise level demands more carbohydrate, increase the CBs™ one at a time. Remember that Carb Booster™ cereal choices are **additional** to cereal at breakfast.

Alcoholic Drinks

½pt beer, lager or dry cider or 1 glass dry wine, or 2 pub measures of spirits, with low-calorie mixers only. Or, save your drinks for one or two nights out. Don't forget, alcohol is not a substitute for water. Top up those fluids!

Breakfasts (choose one each day)

- 2 slices **toast** topped with grilled tomatoes, 1 rasher grilled back or streaky bacon, watercress, cucumber and tomato slices, 1 **apple**, **orange** or **pear**.
- 2 slices **toast** topped with 1 medium egg, poached, grilled tomatoes, watercress, small glass (100ml) **fruit juice**.
- 1 slice **toast** topped with small can (150g) **baked beans**, grilled tomatoes, mushrooms poached in water or stock, watercress, 1 small **banana**.
- 2 **Weetabix** or **Shredded Wheat biscuits**, with milk from allowance, 1 medium **banana**, chopped, a few **raisins**, small glass (100ml) **fruit juice**, 1 carton **low-fat fruit yogurt**.

- **Indian Toast** (recipe, page 142), 1 **apple** or **pear**, 1 small glass (100ml) **fruit juice**.

Light Meals (choose each day)

- Sandwich made with 2 slices **bread** or 1 medium **roll** with 'free' salad and one of the following fillings and accompaniments: either Boots Shapers Ardennes or Peppercorn Pâté, 1 **banana**; or 2 thin slices (50g) lean ham, chicken or other cold meat, 1 **apple**, **pear** or **orange**; or small can (100g) tuna in brine, drained and mixed with lemon juice, 2 **plums** or **satsumas**; or 2tbsps (50g) Light Philadelphia Soft Cheese or other low-fat soft cheese, 1 **apple**, **nectarine** or **peach**; or 1 large (220g) **jacket potato** with any of the toppings on page 151 and a huge 'free' salad, 1 **apple**, **orange** or **peach**.
- 1 chicken drumstick (90g), skin removed, grilled or roasted or 2 thin slices (50g) lean meat with huge 'free' salad, 1 medium **roll**, 1 pot (150g) **Ambrosia Low-Fat Rice Pudding**.
- **Bruschetta with Tomatoes** (recipe, page 166), huge 'free' salad.
- **Mango and Prawns with Melon** (recipe, page 153), huge 'free' salad, 1 medium **roll**, 1 **apple**, **orange** or small **banana**.

Main Meals (choose one each day)

- Large slice **melon**, Lemon Chicken (recipe, page 161), 3tbsps (120g) plain, boiled **rice**, 'free' vegetables and salad, **Pineapple Slices** in Red Wine (recipe, page 184).
- ½ **grapefruit** or medium slice **melon**, 3 thin slices (75g) any lean meat, thin gravy, 'free' vegetables, 2tbsps (60g) **peas**, 1 pot **Ambrosia Low-Fat Rice Pudding**, or 1 **baked apple** with 1tsp clear honey and 1tbsp (25g) **low-fat fruit yogurt**.
- Medium portion (150g) any white fish, grilled, steamed or baked with lemon juice, 'free' vegetables and a little low-fat spread, 1 large (220g) **jacket potato**, 1 **apple** or **orange**.
- **Spaghettini** with Prawns and Garlic (recipe, page 167), huge

'free' salad, 2 scoops vanilla **ice cream** or 2 scoops **fruit sorbet**.

- 1 well-grilled beefburger, grilled tomatoes, 'free' vegetables, small portion (100g) **oven chips**, **Crunchy Fruit Brûlée** (recipe, page 183).
- Any **rice-** or **pasta-based Findus Lean Cuisine** or **Weight Watchers from Heinz** ready-meal with huge portion 'free' salad and vegetables, 1 **apple**, **orange**, **pear** or small **banana**, 1 carton **low-fat fruit yogurt** or 1 pot (150g) **Ambrosia Low-Fat Rice Pudding**, or 2 scoops **fruit sorbet**.

Eating Out

- Indian: Chicken Tikka or Tandoori, plain boiled **rice**, salad.
- Carvery: **melon**, 2 slices (50g) lean roast meat, 1 large (220g) **jacket potato** and plenty of 'free' vegetables.
- Steakhouse: small fillet or rump (115g) steak with 'free' vegetables and salad, **ice cream**.
- Italian (a good choice for exercisers!): **minestrone soup** or mozzarella and tomato salad with basil or Parma ham with **melon**, **pasta with clams** or **tomato sauce**.

The Young Set

As was explained in Chapter Two, children learn their food culture from their parents, friends and at school and it is important that they have a very natural relationship with their food. However, sometimes too much weight is gained in proportion to a child's height and the child may look overweight. This is not the time to panic, but to look again at what they are eating. Is the child eating a varied diet? Are they having fruit and vegetables, or are there too many meals with just chips as an accompaniment to the main item on the plate? Are there no 'set' family meals at certain times, just a constant flow of food?

If too much food is going past those young lips, what can be done? Putting a younger child on a diet is not a good idea as it may make them restrict their food intake too much or develop a poor relationship with food. They may even become 'inhibited' eaters. Changing the pattern of eating or the type of food dished up is the best way forward and will have a longer-term effect. Aiming to hold weight constant while they 'grow into' that weight is ideal and natural. The message, especially about the lifestyle changes for the teen group given below, can be equally applicable to the younger child.

If you are a teenager, or the parent of one, then this section will be very encouraging. Why? Because System S is one eating programme that is recommended for young people who are worried about their weight. It is such a 'normal' and balanced way of eating that it fits into their lifestyle and becomes a blueprint for a lifetime of good nutrition. No foods are considered 'treats' or 'sins', and none are specifically banned on the diet. So, a youngster's relationship with food is a healthy one, with no hangups!

Some people might argue that the word 'diet' should never be uttered in front of an impressionable teenager. Yet, despite all the talk about the dangers of slimming, the fact remains that our young people do need to be helped to eat sensibly for good health. It's too easy to assume that teenagers will eat reasonably well if they are left to their own devices. They won't! Sadly, adequate nutrition information is not always given in schools, and many parents are confused by an over-abundance of conflicting messages given by the food industry, the health organisations and well-meaning journalists.

If you are a chubby teenage boy or girl, you probably get fed up with people telling you that you will 'grow out' of your problems. Yes, you want to shout, but what about now? It is no fun to be the fattest person in the class, to be unable to buy clothes with your pals on a Saturday afternoon because nothing fits, or to be too embarrassed to play sport or take part in school or college activities. The trouble is that all these things also contribute to your weight problem: you start 'comfort-eating' to cheer yourself up when people are rude, go to the fast food joint instead of clothes-shopping with your pals, and munch biscuits while you watch sport on TV! It's a vicious circle.

So, what do you do? First, you can make some very subtle changes in your daily routine to ensure that your general nutrition levels are healthier than they are now. Second, you can follow the diet plan at the end of this section to help you to lose weight sensibly without depriving yourself of the essential nutrients – proteins, fats, carbohydrates, vitamins and minerals – that you need to make sure you develop healthy skin and hair, strong bones and teeth, and the stamina that you need to cope with all the hard work and excitement of your teenage years.

Right, how about those subtle changes? Here is a typical day in the life of Emma, a 16-year-old day school student. Right now she cannot enjoy herself as much as she should because she is 20kg (3st) overweight. Read her timetable, then our comments on just how she can change things to help her get into great shape.

8am Emma gets up, brushes her teeth, dresses and rushes to catch her bus to school. There is no time for breakfast because she is late. She misses the bus anyway, and pops into the store near the bus stop for some crisps and a choc bar.

9am–12noon Lessons are demanding and Emma works very hard. She starts feeling tired at about 11.30am and can feel her concentration slipping. By 11.45am she is very hungry.

12.15pm Lunchtime. Emma has some money to spend in the school canteen or local shops. She is saving up for some new trainers, so she decides to spend half of it on some sweets and a fizzy drink instead of having a proper meal. Going without dinner will, she thinks, help her to lose some weight.

2–3.30pm Art and drama this afternoon. Emma likes both subjects, but she is still feeling sleepy. So, when there's a break between lessons, she goes to the tuckshop and buys a doughnut. She feels a bit better.

4.30pm A pal's mum takes Emma and a friend to a burger bar. Emma is ravenous and tucks into a burger, but leaves the chips (weight-watching, again). The burger contains plenty of calories (over 500), and 33g of fat, but somehow, afterwards, she is still hungry.

6pm Emma eats dinner with her family. She picks at her meal, because her mum and dad have already told her how worried they are about her weight.

8pm She goes to her room to do homework. While she is working, she nibbles a couple of chocolate biscuits taken from the secret supply she keeps at the bottom of her wardrobe.

10pm Bedtime.

During her day, Emma is always reacting to situations instead of initiating them. Although her school and homework routine can't be changed, there are other ways she can 'do her own thing', especially where food is concerned. Although she wants, desperately, to shed some weight, everything she does at the moment is guaranteed to prevent her from achieving that aim. Here's how she can change things.

Instead of getting up late, she should set the alarm for 7.30, and eat breakfast – cereal, fruit and a yogurt, perhaps. She could also prepare a packed lunch to take to school.

There is nothing wrong with nibbling a few sweets on the bus – in fact, if she follows the eating plan below she can choose 10 Paynes Poppets or a fun size Mars Bar from the Carbohydrate Boosters™ on pages 61–2. At lunchtime, she can settle down with her own packed spread (a sandwich, some crisps, fruit and a drink, perhaps) in the canteen or playground.

After school, she could suggest to her friend and her friend's mum that they go for a walk in the park or around the shops instead of eating burgers. At home, she can sit down to a meal (including dessert) with the family without having to feel guilty about enjoying it.

In the evening, she should take fruit to her room to munch while she works, plus another Carb Booster™ if she is following the diet. Half-way through her homework session, she can have an exercise break – working out to pop music or a video. As her confidence improves, she can include more exercise in her daily routine.

Here are ten tips to help you (and Emma!) shape up.

1. Help your mum and dad with the shopping. If you go around the shops together, you can pick out the foods that you enjoy, and are healthy. Discuss your likes and dislikes; offer to do some of the food preparation.

2. Eat breakfast. It is important to have a good meal before you face the day. It doesn't have to be complicated, or even cooked. (Although you will probably enjoy recipes like Indian Toast (recipe, page 142) and Saucy Beans on Toast (recipe, page 145).

3. Eat regularly. Going for long periods without food won't help you slim, it will simply make you ravenous which could lead to a chocolate biscuit binge later on.

4. Have sweets and sweet puds when you fancy them. Don't think of them as 'bad' – no food is, in itself, bad for you. Every food can have its place in a healthy diet.

5. Always keep some fruit (and a Carb Booster™ if you are following the eating plan) in your bag or rucksack, then you can beat the energy-gap between lessons without spending money in the tuckshop.

6. If people tease you about your size, stay cool. They are stuck with their big noses or stringy hair, you can improve your shape. Choose friends who value you for yourself, not those who judge you by what you look like.

7. Find an exercise activity that you really enjoy: for example, dancing, yoga, riding, skating or bowling.

8. Eat with the family. If your brothers, sisters or even your parents make pointed remarks about the amount of food you put on your plate have a quiet word with your mum or dad about it. Tell them how much it hurts and ask them to stop.

9. Be open about your eating habits. If you fancy a choc bar in front of the telly, have one. If you go to your room and eat secretly, you will feel guilty and will probably have two choc bars instead.

10. Be independent. Don't let TV advertisements, supermarket bosses or junk food moguls tell you what to eat and drink. *You* decide!

Teenage Plan

This is a plan which allows 1800 Cals daily and 250g carbohydrate. It is suitable for teenagers who are worried about their weight. There is an extra milk allowance and teenagers should top up their vegetables as well to ensure they get plenty of vitamins for healthy growth and development.

Daily Allowance

430ml (¾pt) semi-skimmed milk for tea, coffee and cereals, unlimited water and mineral water and diet soft drinks (go easy).

Free Vegetables

Choose from the list on page 56.

Carb Boosters™

Choose **three** from the lists on pages 61–2. Remember that Carb Booster™ cereal choices are **additional** to cereal at breakfast.

Breakfasts (choose one each day)

- 2 **Weetabix** or **2 Shredded Wheat biscuits**, with milk from allowance, 1 slice **toast** with 1tsp **jam** or **marmalade**, 1 **apple**, **orange**, **pear** or small **banana**.
- Sandwich made with 2 slices **bread**, spread with Marmite or mild mustard, with one of the following fillings and accompaniments: either 1 rasher well-grilled crispy bacon, tomatoes, watercress; or Kraft Cheese Triangle, tomato, cucumber; or small can (100g) tuna in brine, drained and mixed with lemon juice; and either 1 **apple**, **pear** or small **banana** and small glass (100ml) **fruit juice**.
- 2 slices **toast** topped with small can (150g) **baked beans**, grilled tomatoes, watercress, small glass (100ml) **fruit juice**.
- **Indian Toast** (recipe, page 142), small glass (100ml) **fruit juice**, 1 carton **low-fat fruit yogurt** or an **additional CB™**.
- 7tbsps (45g) **sweetened cereal**, with milk from allowance, 1 slice **toast**, 1tsp **jam**.

Choose either a packed lunch or a snack meal each day.

Packed Lunches (for school or work)

- 2 slices **bread** or 1 medium **roll**, with one of the following fillings and accompaniments plus plenty of 'free' salad and vegetables: either Shippams Sardine and Tomato Spread or Mild Vegetable Curry Spread, with watercress, plus 1 carton **low-fat fruit yogurt**; or 1 slice (25g) roast chicken, lean ham, or pork (no skin or fat), 1 **apple**, 1 packet low-fat crisps; or 2tbsps (30g) **Heinz Sandwich Spread**, 1 large **banana**.
- **Pasta Salad** (recipe, page 149), large 'free' salad, 1 mug slimmer's soup, any flavour, 1 **orange** or 2 **satsumas**.
- 1 pot Golden Wonder Pot Light **pot noodles**, 2 medium **rolls** (add 'free' salad to one and 1tbsp **jam** or **marmalade** to the other), 1 **apple**, **orange** or **pear**.
- 1 medium **roll** or small (75g) **pitta bread** with filling of salad and can (100g) tuna in brine, drained and mixed with lemon juice, 2 **jaffa cakes**, a few **grapes** or 1 **satsuma**.

Snack Meals (eat at home or at a friend's house)

- 1 medium beefburger or veggieburger (100g), grilled, **bun**, salad, 2tsps relish or tomato sauce, huge 'free' salad, 1 large **banana**.
- Large (220g) **jacket potato** with any of the fillings on page 151, huge mixed 'free' salad, 1 carton **low-fat fruit yogurt**.
- 2 well-grilled low-fat sausages, 'free' salad and vegetables, 2 slices **bread** or 1 medium **roll**, 1 **apple** and **orange**.
- 2 slices **toast** topped with 1 medium egg, poached, with small can (150g) **baked beans** and grilled tomatoes, 1 **apple**, **pear** or medium **banana**.

Main Meals

- **Boston Baked Beans** (recipe, page 160), 1 **roll** or slice of **bread**, 'free' vegetables and salad, 1 medium portion (140g) canned **fruit in syrup**, 1tbsp **low-fat fruit yogurt**.
- 1 slice **melon**, 3 slices (75g) lean roast meat, thin gravy, large (220g) **jacket potato**, 'free' vegetables, 1tbsp (30g) **peas**, 1 carton **low-fat fruit yogurt**.
- **Oodles of Noodles Stir-Fry** (recipe, page 163), huge mixed salad from 'free' list, 1 medium **banana**, 2 **jaffa cakes**.
- Birds Eye Cod Steak in **Harvest Crumb** or 2 Salmon Fish Cakes in **Wholemeal Crumb**, or Cod Steak in Mushroom or Parsley Sauce, small portion (100g) **oven chips**, grilled tomatoes, 1 medium **roll**, bowl (180g) **fruit-flavoured jelly**.
- Matthews Turkey Burger or Golden Drummer, small portion (100g) oven chips, 2tbsps (60g) **peas**, huge portion 'free' vegetables or salad, 1 **meringue nest** with medium portion (90g) **can of raspberries in syrup**.
- Spanish Chicken (recipe page 179), 'free' vegetables, 3tbsps (120g) plain, boiled **rice**, 1 medium **roll**, 1 **apple**, **orange** or small **banana**.

NOTE: if you are taking part in a school match, have an extra CB™ on the day.

CHAPTER SEVEN

System S Case Histories

During the twelve-week System S study, our thirty 'guinea pigs' tested a revolutionary new way of eating. Not surprisingly, they found the food plans rather unusual. Most had followed other diets which banned sweet foods or allowed them only as 'treats' or 'sins'; it was quite a shock to read a diet sheet that actually told them they *must* eat things like sugar-coated cereals, chocolate bars and slices of gateau. They felt that the diet must somehow be 'naughty', even though the menus also contained plenty of foods perceived as 'healthy', including lean meat, fish, vegetables, fruits and complex carbohydrate foods like bread, potatoes and pasta.

Those who had a 'sweet tooth' were pleased – although very surprised – that they would at last be able to eat sucrose-containing foods without feeling guilty. However, some were also fearful that the sudden green light would set them off into a downward spiral of sweet bingeing (which didn't, in fact, happen!).

Pat Aiton, who lost 8kg (18½lb) during the twelve weeks and now weighs a trim 60kg (9st 5lb) was delighted that she could, at last, eat chocolate openly: 'Before starting the diet, I nibbled chocolate secretly – hiding the wrappers down the back of the sofa,' she says. 'It was such a relief to munch my way through a chocolate biscuit or bar of chocolate without having to hide it away. I'm sure that's why I enjoy this new way of eating so much.'

Those with a 'savoury' tooth, who listed such things as pizzas, crisps and chips as their 'food weaknesses', were somewhat resistant to the whole idea of eating a choc bar or bowl of Crunchy Nut Cornflakes at all. After all, if they didn't enjoy sweet foods, what was the point of having them? Surely, they would lose weight more quickly if they ignored the Carb Booster™ list? Once Professor de Looy had explained to the group that the Carb Boosters™ were vital to make the diet work, our volunteers were happy to eat them. Deborah Handy, who lost 7kg (15lb) during the trial and now weighs in at 75kg (11st 11lb), found it hard to believe that she was supposed to eat chocolate-coated biscuits and sweet cereals every single day.

'My problem has always been over-indulging in high-fat savoury foods like pizzas – but I could never eat one piece, it always had to be three or four, and the more cheese on top the better' she says. 'So, eating sweet foods took quite a bit of getting used to. Now, System S has become a way of life. I can order a pizza for the family, and eat just one slice instead of three without bothering. I'm used to having my Carb Boosters™ (I generally choose chocolate biscuits) during coffee breaks and thoroughly enjoy them.'

Debbie's experience illustrates well the effect that the diet has on savoury snack lovers who gained weight because they ate too many crisps, pizzas and other takeaway meals which are high in fat and calories. Once the Carb Boosters™ are included in their diet, they just don't fancy so many chips or those extra slices of pizza that pile on the pounds. So, they lose weight.

Are there any overweight people who would *not* be able to follow System S successfully?

Some of the 'guinea pigs' in our trial did have reservations. Here are some of their observations, recorded during a discussion session after the trial ended:

Questioner: Did the diet work for you?
First Slimmer: I'm dieting on and off all the time. Night time's the worst, when I pick and eat chocolate. I stored my sweet foods up for the evening, but I found I wanted to pig out. I tried it for three months, but then switched to a different version, without the Carbohydrate Boosters™.

SECOND SLIMMER: I have a big problem with blood sugar and it goes in a monthly cycle as well. If I'm allowed any sugar at all, I have to have more and more. I lost any form of structure with the diet. It blew my control. I would prefer to be on a diet with no chocolate or sweets at all.

Third Slimmer: I feel more confident if I'm not allowed any sugary foods, which I think of as treats. If I get fed up, I think one more treat won't hurt. If I have one chocolate biscuit, I'll eat the whole packet.

First Slimmer: I have a real chocolate addiction, it's like alcoholism. Sometimes, it's so bad that I shake.

Third Slimmer: I do try to have breakfast, and having cereal plus toast and jam filled me up. However, I didn't feel any more full with System S than on The Fatfield Diet.

Professor Anne de Looy says:

'These three slimmers are all being very honest and are expressing real concerns. We have all been there.

'The first slimmer has a problem with "picking" at food in the evenings. Certainly, evenings are a difficult time, because that is when we relax and can also become bored. If the day has been busy then we are looking for something to do and eating is just as good as anything else. If you are at a loose end in the evening, then try eating low-calorie foods: a bowl of microwaved popcorn is a good choice. Or, have a box of ready-prepared fresh vegetables in the fridge.

'We turn to biscuits and other nibbles because they require no effort to prepare, but a bowl of tasty vegetables, cut into bite-size pieces or strips is just like having a "convenience food", but with very few of the calories. For many people, however, this is just not the same as having something sweet. One of the many good things about System S, is that you can use a Carbohydrate Booster™ as your evening snack. You could also save your bread or potato to eat in the evening. My fridge has cold boiled or baked potatoes in it which I often have at night.

'In the first slimmer, it is also possible to recognise the "inhibited"

eater, the type of slimmer which I mentioned in Chapter Two. Once he or she starts eating, then off they go! Remember, you don't have to do this. However, it does take time to reverse the beliefs you hold and it won't be done in a few weeks. Returning to a diet that is tested and works for that individual is important, but I hope that over the course of the next year she learns to live with her food. If she can practise having some Carbohydrate Boosters™, they will help her learn control.

'The second slimmer also has a tendency towards "inhibited eating", but she also recognises that she has a monthly cycle. Carbohydrate comes into our body in two ways – the sugary kind which is sweet and the starchy kind, not sweet, which we find in rice, pasta, potatoes and bread. On System S, you get both kinds. Sugar carbohydrate can be absorbed more quickly than the starchy kind, but the absorption rate depends on the overall combination of the diet. For some people, a diet that is richer in the starchy form of carbohydrate may be easier to handle at certain times of the month. It may be the week before the cravings start that the difference is made, so it is well worth experimenting. This slimmer has made a very positive choice.

'The third slimmer is a typical "inhibited" eater. She is going to do something about it by returning, quite sensibly, to a tried and tested diet that has worked for her, in this case The Fatfield Diet. Great, but at some point she will still have to confront her beliefs about her eating habits if she is to have long-term success. However, now might not be the time. In cases like this, it is very useful to have the support of diet counsellors and the encouragement to change. These are very positive events. She didn't give up!

For the vast majority of overweight people, though, System S is nothing short of miraculous and is hugely enjoyable to follow.

Here are some inspiring stories from six slimmers who took part in the twelve-week trial, with Professor de Looy's comments.

Slimmer One

Name: Pat Aiton

Occupation: Voluntary worker

Starting Weight: 73kg (11st 6½lb)

Weight Now: 60kg (9st 5lb)

Age: 51

Height: 1.6m (5ft 4in)

Weight After 12 Weeks:
64kg (10st 2lb)

Energetic Pat is now so slim and fit that she feels ten years younger than she did before starting System S. She is an enthusiastic Line Dancing fan, and sometimes goes to her classes five or six times a week. She also teaches at her local village hall. 'A year ago, that would have been out of the question,' she says. 'I felt extremely uncomfortable and looked dreadful in jeans. Now, I enjoy wearing the whole outfit – tight, size 12 jeans, boots, fringed shirt, boots and hat. It is great fun.'

Pat, who is retired but does a lot of voluntary work for her local church, blames her hectic social life for her weight-gain last year. 'My husband and I have no children so we have a very relaxed lifestyle,' she says. 'We go to lots of parties, dinners and receptions.'

Before she started the diet, Pat was always first in the queue for sausage rolls and nibbles, and loved the sweets and cakes. 'Chocolate was my passion,' she says. 'I'm afraid I became quite secretive about my chocolate-eating habit. One day I was caught out when the doorbell rang and I quickly stuffed my chocolate wrapper down the back of the sofa before getting up to open the door. The dog sniffed out the wrapper and brought it to the door in his mouth. My husband laughed heartily but I felt very silly indeed.'

When she started the diet, Pat was afraid that she would be tempted to eat more Carb Boosters™ than she should. 'I thought I would cut out chocolate completely and get my sucrose from the sweet drinks like lemonade that are allowed on the diet,' she says. 'As I began to feel more confident, and the weight started to drop off, I included a low-calorie chocolate bar every day.

'Amazingly, I had no urge to eat more than one. I think

there are probably two reasons for this. First, I felt so full up on the diet that I didn't crave my usual chocolate "fix", and second, I was confident that I could eat my daily chocolate ration openly, in front of my husband, John. Interestingly, he is also more controlled about his own sweet-eating. We are both more honest and able to be truthful about the foods we enjoy.'

Pat is now able to wear fashionable clothes, and has put all her old size 16 outfits away in a cupboard. 'I certainly haven't cut back on my social life,' she says. 'But, these days, I can face a party buffet spread without having to tuck into every single goodie on display. I am quite satisfied with a small plateful, instead of a huge mound of food.'

Professor Anne de Looy says:

'People with a hectic lifestyle often eat food "on the go". This often spells disaster for those who find it difficult to control their food intake because they simply can't remember what they've eaten. Eating out can also be a problem because the buffet table is groaning under the weight of "party foods" which in our culture often means high-fat food. Somehow a plate of vegetables or fresh fruit looks much less luxurious and appetising when it is next to a plate of vol-au-vents or gateaux. After all, when you are out socialising, your host and hostess like to "treat" you. In our culture, we all share a conception about what is a treat and then enjoy feeling naughty when we eat it. So, you'll have noticed that we have removed the word "treat" from the diets in this book. All foods can be special, but we need to savour them.

'Pat eats her chocolate or party foods to please herself. She doesn't need to fill up her plate or eat chocolate secretly because she feels confident in the pleasure she derives from food and life and that's often linked with self-worth and self-knowledge. Pat knows what suits her. She has discovered that being honest to yourself is very important when you are faced with daily food choices. Chocolate and other foods can be included without any problems, when you are in control.'

Slimmer Two

Name: Muriel Farr

Occupation: Retired colour consultant

Starting Weight: 65kg (10st 3lb)

Weight Now: 57kg (9st)

Age: 61

Height: 1.6m (5ft 2in)

Weight After 12 Weeks: 60kg (9st 7lb)

Elegant Muriel was never hugely overweight, but she gained 4.5kg (10lb) last year after her daughter's wedding. 'It was held in a Scottish castle,' she says. 'I did all the flower arrangements, and the whole thing was quite wonderful, although very exhausting. I bought a beautiful new cream outfit which looked great on the day. Afterwards, I just relaxed and the pounds piled on. Six weeks later, I was horrified when I couldn't get into my outfit.'

Muriel has a sweet tooth, so when she heard about the System S trial, she was keen to take part. 'I decided to have chocolate fudge bars as my Carb Boosters™,' she says. 'I bought my supply every week, and kept it in a cupboard in the kitchen which I use for storing kitchen utensils. I don't open it every day, so I knew I wouldn't have to keep looking at the fudge!

'I needn't have worried. After I'd been following the diet for a few days, I really didn't feel like eating a lot of sweets and I stopped craving fatty foods, too. Things like grated cheese on the top of soup, butter on bread and on potatoes seemed so greasy somehow. I just didn't want them any more. I also choose more vegetable dishes these days. For instance, if there is a list of starters on a restaurant menu, I will always go for the vegetable soup or the melon, rather than the fatty pâté. Not because I'm watching my weight, but because that is what I fancy eating.'

Muriel and her husband Malcolm, a retired pharmacist, do a lot of travelling, and she was worried that tempting foreign dishes would ruin her diet. 'Right in the middle of the trial, we went away to Tenerife for a week,' she says. 'I managed to stick to the plan really well and only put on a couple of pounds, which I then lost very quickly. Since the end of the trial, the diet plan has become a way of life. I am happy with my size now, although I would like to lose just a little more weight.'

Her experience as a colour consultant has given Muriel a brilliant eye for fashion, and she is now able to indulge her passion for designer clothes. 'The best thing is that I can now wear my beautiful mother-of-the-bride outfit once more.'

Professor Anne de Looy says:

'Isn't it interesting that once you know you can have something, it becomes less important in your life? Muriel knew the chocolate was there in her cupboard, and could have been eaten, yet didn't succumb. Many of our System S group saved up their alcohol allowance to have at the weekend. If you know something is there and can be taken at any time, it is often very reassuring. Again, I wonder if that says something about feeling in control. Yet, we all seem to exist in a permanent 'caveman' state. The "don't-know-where-the-next-meal-is-coming-from-and-therefore-I-must-eat-it-now" syndrome.

'Muriel has relaxed about her food. Even after her holiday, she simply reorganised herself and lost those gained pounds. She's also no longer yearning after the taste of fatty foods. Her taste-buds have been retrained – or is it her mind? Or is it possibly the fact that carbohydrate in her diet is more satisfying. There is no one answer for Muriel. The diet has become her way of life.'

Slimmer Three

Name: Deborah Handy

Occupation: Housewife

Starting Weight: 83kg (13st 1lb)

Weight Now: 70kg (11st)

Age: 33

Height: 1.7m (5ft 7in)

Weight After 12 Weeks:
76kg (12st)

Tall, attractive Deborah is a self-confessed 'yo-yo' dieter who has tried lots of different slimming club diets and faddy regimes, including living on milkshake drinks and eggs! Until now, she has never managed to reach a 'happy' weight or find an eating pattern which she could actually stick to. Now, after following System S successfully, she has kept her weight at a steady 70kg (11st) for six months, and feels confident that she will maintain her shapely new size 14 figure.

I gained weight after the birth of each of my three children,' she says. 'My highest ever weight was 87kg (13st 10lb). That was last summer. I would join a slimming club, lose weight quickly, then long for a savoury treat like a pizza or a spicy takeaway. We would order three 12-inch pizzas between the five of us and I would eat at least four or five slices.'

A week before starting the diet trial, Debbie felt that she had lost the whole slimming plot and was about to give up. 'I actually ate 17 slices of bread and butter in one day,' she says. 'Goodness knows why. Then I heard that Professor de Looy and Sally Ann Voak were looking for volunteers to try System S, and I decided to sign up. I had nothing to lose.'

She started the trial feeling very negative about eating the Carb Boosters™. 'I didn't really fancy them, but decided to have the chocolate biscuits with my coffee in the mornings and my tea in the afternoons or just before bed-time,' she says. 'I soon got used to the taste of something sweet, and now enjoy my biscuits very much indeed. We buy most things in bulk, but I buy my chocolate biscuits every day. The children have one each for their packed lunch and I have mine. It's nice to know that we all eat the same thing.'

'One of the big bonuses of the diet is that I never, ever feel hungry these days. The meals are easy to prepare, and my tastebuds have changed. I eat things like fish which I had never fancied before.

Her husband Les, forty-two years old, works shifts as a careworker at a special needs school, so Deborah often has to prepare meals in relays – for her children Rachel, twelve, Victoria, ten, and Steven, eight, for herself, and then for Les. 'In the past, I would have been nibbling away while I cooked,' she says. 'But, once I got into the swing of the diet, I found I could prepare my own meal in about 10 minutes. Now, I really enjoy my food and don't want to snack. I am particularly pleased that I have lost a lot of inches – about 18½ in total.'

Debbie now has the confidence to wear a swimsuit, and goes to her local pool three times a week. Her children and husband are thrilled, too. 'It is like being a new person,' she says. 'I feel so much healthier, and I love dressing up instead of wearing the same old dreary "uniform" of leggings and sloppy sweater. Recently, I went out in new suit with a long skirt and jacket and met one of the mums from school, who didn't recognise me.'

Professor Anne de Looy says:
'Deborah has really made this diet her own and she fits it into her lifestyle. Buying chocolate biscuits every day works for her and she knows that. She is in control of that part of her life and has managed to work out a routine which suits her busy household. By cooking herself a quick, yet nutritious meal she can satisfy her hunger and not pick or nibble while coping with the rest of the family. This is a really important change which will help Deborah. We all get hungry and the easiest thing to eat is the food or drink item that is right in front of our noses. Unfortunately, it is usually not an apple or a stick of carrot.

'With System S you can find snacks which are around and make them part of your eating regime, such as a finger of fudge or a biscuit. Because they are part of the diet, you can be confident and relaxed about eating them. These Carbohydrate Boosters™ are important as they speak about who you are: a normal, valued human being. The recipes are also to boost the carbohydrate content of the diet, which is recommended by all health experts. High carbohydrate meals are satisfying, nourishing and will provide all the energy she needs for activities such as swimming.

'Debbie has seen a boost in her confidence which comes with weight loss. She has more energy and drive which, of course, is good news for keeping off the pounds. Activity is vital for regulating body weight and also for cardiovascular health. This is a real success story, not just because of the weight-loss but because of all the other things going on in her life.'

Slimmer Four

Name: Denise James   **Age:** 37

Occupation: Voluntary worker   **Height:** 1.6m (5ft 4in)

Starting Weight: 74kg (11st 9lb)   **Weight After 12 Weeks:**

Weight Now: 68kg (10st 12½lb)   68kg (10st 12½lb)

Pretty Denise found it difficult to get used to eating sweet foods at first, especially when her family expressed their amazement at her new 'slimming' diet. 'I chose the Crunchy Nut Corn Flakes for breakfast, and as a second Carb Booster™ in the evenings and also ate a mini Mars Bar during the day,' she says. 'My two children were shocked. My son said "Mum, how can you lose weight if you eat so many sweet things?"'

Denise works hard as a voluntary worker for her local church and also runs a toddlers' group and Sunday school. Although she has always had a pleasantly rounded figure, her weight crept up after having her children. She lost 20kg (3st) at a slimming club, then hurt her back and the weight piled on again. 'I got a real shock when I stepped on the scales and found how much I weighed,' she says. 'It was very daunting to realise that I had to start all over again. But once I committed myself to taking part in the diet trial, I decided I would stick to it – despite my misgivings about the strange foods!' She is now very glad she did. 'Although I had to force myself to eat the chocolate bar during the day, I really enjoyed having my sweet cereal snack in the evening,' she says. 'It felt wicked. It was a lovely way to finish the day.'

Denise is still adjusting to the diet, but even though she has slipped off the programme slightly, her weight has maintained. One of the problems is that she still thinks her Carb Boosters™ are 'wicked'. An important part of the philosophy of the plan is that no food should be considered wicked or even a 'treat'. All foods, even those containing fat, have their part to play in a balanced, tasty, palatable eating plan. For slimmers like Denise who have been indoctrinated in the old theory that certain things are 'naughty' or 'baddies', it takes some getting used to!

'I know it works, but it still doesn't feel quite right to eat the sweet foods, probably because I have always been taught that they are unhealthy and bad for your teeth,' says Denise. 'But I would like to lose another stone this year, and I am determined to carry on with System S. I think this is a diet that people with a lot of weight to lose would find very easy, especially if they are fed up with yo-yo dieting and following slimming club rules. Despite my own problems with accepting the sweet foods, I also approve of the fact that they are not taboo. I teach my four-year-old daughter and the children at my toddlers' group that they should enjoy a variety of foods, not just a few.'

Professor Anne de Looy says:

'Isn't it interesting how much our friends and family influence our food intake? In fact it is one of the major influences. We eat to please people and we eat things to spite people, but how often do we eat to really please ourselves? To feel good about ourselves? System S forces you to confront the prejudices and other thoughts we and our families hold, and that is a good thing.

Denise found that by enjoying herself, especially with the cereal snack in the evening, she could cope with the diet. 'It felt wicked. It was a lovely way to finish the day,' she says. It's strange that we should think of food as wicked, when it isn't wicked at all. That is simply our perception, reinforced by others. If Denise had just come out of a long illness and lost 3 stone, I am sure her family would be saying 'eat, eat, eat'. Food wouldn't be wicked then.

So, looking at food as a vital part of your life where no individual food is good or bad, healthy or unhealthy is a good place to start. It is how these foods are put together in the diet, how frequently they are eaten and how much is eaten which matters. We all need to adopt a less judgmental attitude if we are to live comfortably in our food environment.

In Denise's home, where a four-and-a-half-year-old lives, there are bound to be lots of different foods coming and going. Denise has to cope with this environment. Of course, she can manipulate what food is bought, but she can't always do so for her daughter as she grows up and goes to school. So, getting her daughter to accept a wide range of foods with a high emphasis on fruit and vegetables but acknowledging that sweet foods can also be eaten is very important. If Denise can maintain her weight loss, then I think there is no greater testament to her success. There are very few people who would fail to lose weight with System S, but the real test is whether the diet has enabled people to reorganise their eating patterns to maintain that loss. A balanced approach to your food environment is the very best way to start.'

Slimmer Five

Name: Susan Burnip **Age:** 42
Occupation: Housewife **Height:** 1.5m (4ft 11in)
Starting Weight: 66kg (10st 4½lb) **Weight After 12 Weeks:**
Weight Now: 58kg (9st 2lb) 60kg (9st 6½lb)

Tiny Sue gained 13kg (2st) after having her third child, who is now two and a half. 'I'd suffered major health problems before the pregnancy and then had a hysterectomy a year after my daughter's birth,' she says. 'I have two other children age seventeen and fifteen, so I'm afraid my eating habits became extremely erratic and unhealthy. I'd nibble chips between meals and prepare fast, easy things instead of balanced dishes. It was terribly difficult because I was so busy and very tired all the time. My ankles started to swell up and I was worried about my health.'

After losing 5.5kg (12lb) on a slimming club diet, Sue found that the flab was starting to creep back on again, so she volunteered to try the new diet plan. 'I was still at the stage where I hid my tummy under a huge baggy top and wore leggings underneath,' she says. 'I don't have a sweet tooth, but I thought the diet sounded interesting so I decided to give it a try.'

Like all our volunteers, Sue was given a diet sheet with a good choice of meals, plus the Free Vegetables, Carb Boosters™ and Alcohol allowance, and she was told to write down everything she ate and drank each day. 'I had bran flakes and skimmed milk for breakfast, with a slice of toast and jam to follow,' she says. 'It's interesting because I had never ever eaten jam on toast before. I had always spread plenty of butter on my breakfast toast ration. Now, I find that the sweet taste of jam is far more refreshing.'

'Lunch was a tuna or low-fat cheese spread sandwich with plenty of salad, followed by a fruit yogurt or piece of fruit, and we always had a cooked supper such as a chicken casserole with new potatoes and lots of other vegetables. My husband and children could eat exactly the same as me with extra complex carbohydrate foods like bread, potatoes and pasta. My husband, Alan, has a physically demanding job and is 1.8m (6ft) tall, so he has a hearty appetite, but he was quite satisfied with my diet foods.'

Sue noticed a dramatic change in her body shape during the twelve-week trial period, despite the fact that she took no additional exercise. 'My waistline virtually disappeared when I had my daughter, so it was wonderful to see it reappearing again,' she says. 'I lost 10cm (4in) off my bustline, 15cm (6in) off my waist and 8cm (3in) off my hips. Even the tops of my thighs shrank by 5cm (2in) each, and I lost the same amount of flab from the tops of my arms. It was quite remarkable.' Sue's older children Alan, seventeen, and Laura, fifteen, are very complimentary about their 'new' mum. 'They tell me I look gorgeous, which is wonderful,' she says. 'I certainly do feel like a new woman.'

Professor de Looy says:

'Like Sue, many women find that they can trace their weight gain back to a pregnancy or pregnancies. Nature prepares women's bodies very well to nurture a foetus for nine whole months. Unfortunately, in our society, we don't quite need all the additional fat afterwards! Slimming clubs can work wonders, but then it is up to the individual to maintain the weight loss. This is the big problem.

Too often, we go back to the same lifestyle as before, unaware that to maintain weight you need to think even more carefully about how you put your food life together because you are on your own. There is no weekly weigh-in or encouragement from a sympathetic (or unsympathetic!) slimming club leader. So, Susan has done well to recognise that she needed to keep up the pressure and get the reassurance which comes from regular attendance at a club. She has also turned her diet pattern into one that suits the whole family. This is very important because the principles of System S are ones advocated by health professionals. Eat lots of vegetables, complex carbohydrate and fruit . . . and don't be shy about sweet foods either. The whole family can eat better and fill up on the high carbohydrate foods such as bread, pasta and potatoes. This sounds like a very supportive family which I am sure helped Susan to feel like a new woman.'

Slimmer Six

Name: Lorraine Mitchell   **Age:** 35

Occupation: Housewife   **Height:** 1.6m (5ft 4in)

Starting Weight: 66kg (10st 7lb)   **Weight After 12 Weeks:**

Weight Now: 57kg (9st)   61kg (9st 10lb)

Bubbly Lorraine thought she would never, ever be able to eat another bowl of sugar-coated Frosties, until she started System S and was told to eat *two* bowls containing 7 tablespoons in each bowl, every single day.

'I always thought sweet cereals were terribly bad for you and very fattening,' she says. 'And, as I was constantly struggling to lose weight, they were one food that I avoided, even though I loved them. Now, I wonder why I worried so much.'

Lorraine, who has four children aged between three and twelve, was a very slim teenager, but gained weight after each pregnancy. 'I weighed only about 53kg (8st 4lb) when I was eighteen,' she says. 'But when I had my third child, Karl, my weight shot up to 80kg (12½st), and I found it very difficult to shift it afterwards.'

After having her fourth baby, Becky, who is now three, Lorraine did manage to slim down to 67kg (10½st), but still felt large. 'I hated those awful rolls of flab above my jeans,' she says.

'Although my husband, Andy, said I was "cuddly", I still felt fat.

When she volunteered to be a 'guinea pig', Lorraine was astonished when she was given her diet sheet – and saw the Frosties on the list of Carb Boosters™. 'I thought it was a mistake,' she says. 'When I found out that I could really eat them, I had to "give myself permission" to eat them, which sounds crazy, I know.'

Once she had got used to the diet, Lorraine loved it. 'It is now a way of life for me, ' she says. 'I have lost 8cm (3in) off my waistline and 5cm (2in) each off my bust and hips. I can wear swimsuits with confidence and go to the baths three times a week. I do 10 minutes of water aerobics to warm up, then swim 40 lengths. Before starting the diet, I had so little energy. Now, I feel I can do anything.'

'My little daughter summed it up when she came into the bathroom and saw me, naked, in the tub. She said. "Eee, mummy, you're lovely and slim lying down in the bath. Where's your big tummy gone?" These days, I feel pretty slim standing up, too!'

Professor Anne de Looy says:
'Our muscles need both carbohydrate and fat for energy. As most people know, fat is in almost unlimited supply in our bodies, but the carbohydrate needs replacing every day because we store so little. By emphasising the need to increase carbohydrate with System S, our muscles will have plenty of fuel and, as in the case of Lorraine, they can and should be able to be worked hard. The exercise programme will help Lorraine to maintain her weight loss as well as keep her body well-honed. Unfairly, sweet foods have really had a lot of bad publicity with respect to their energy or calorie value. Sugar has half the energy of fat, weight for weight. So, to think that all sweet foods are fattening is inaccurate, and does them a disservice. A slice of bread and jam contains about 100 Cals, but a slice of bread and butter or margarine contains about 160. Toast is probably even higher as the fat melts and is sucked up into the bread like a sponge. Foods which are high in fat are therefore those to be careful with but, just like Lorraine, we need to eat a variety of foods, which is what System S is all about.'

PART TWO

The Recipes

(v) = suitable for vegetarians

Breakfasts

Here are six delicious recipes for breakfasts. They are all quick to make (the night before, if you are really rushed off your feet in the mornings), and will set you, and the family, up for the day.

Lentil and Lime Kedgeree

This is a new twist on an old favourite. The classic kedgeree ingredients of cooked smoked haddock, hard-boiled eggs and rice are given extra interest with the addition of lime pickle, lemon juice and lentils.

100g (4oz) brown rice
100g (4oz) lentils
3 hard-boiled eggs, shelled and roughly chopped
1tbsp (15ml) lime pickle
400g (1lb) smoked haddock, cooked, flaked and kept hot
1tbsp (15ml) lemon or lime juice and fresh parsley to garnish

1. Cook the rice in plenty of boiling water for about 20 minutes until tender but with 'bite' appeal. Strain and keep warm.
2. Meanwhile, put the lentils in a large pan of cold water, bring to the boil and simmer gently for about 10–15 minutes, until softened but not mushy.
3. Mix together the rice, lentils, eggs, lime pickle and flaked haddock, sprinkle with lemon or lime juice and garnish with chopped parsley. Serve immediately.

Serves: 4
Per portion: Calories 297, Protein 33.5g, Fat 7g, Carbohydrate 29g, Fibre 1g.

Indian Toast (v)

Fancy something hot and spicy for breakfast? This recipe is just
what you need to get you going on a cold winter's morning.
Serve it with some chilled grapefruit juice or a crunchy apple.

100g (4oz) grated Edam or other hard cheese
2tbsps (2 x 15ml) sweet chutney
1tsp (15ml) curry powder
4 tomatoes
4 large slices wholemeal bread

1. Mix the cheese, chutney and curry powder into a thick paste.
Slice the tomatoes.
2. Grill the bread on both sides and then cover one side with
tomatoes and the cheese mixture. Place under the grill for
2–3 minutes until bubbly.

Serves: 4
Per portion: Calories 113, Protein 4g, Fat 2g,
Carbohydrate 21g, Fibre 3g.

Fruity Oats (v)

This has to be tasted to be believed! The combination of rolled oats, citrus fruit and honey is guaranteed to wake up the whole family. You do have to remember to soak the oats in water overnight, but the effort is well worthwhile.

4tbsps (4 x 15ml) rolled oats soaked overnight in just enough water to cover
2 grapefruit (grate a little of the rind)
2 oranges (grate a little of the rind)
150ml (¼pt) natural low-fat yogurt
1tsp clear honey

1. Mix the oats with the yogurt, honey and a little grated orange and grapefruit rind.

2. Peel and segment the oranges and grapefruit, divide between four dishes and spoon the honey and oatmeal mixture on top.

Serves: 4
Per portion: Calories 113, Protein 4g, Fat 2g, Carbohydrate 21g, Fibre 3g.

Smoked Salmon Scramble

This very special 'brunch' version of scrambled eggs, can be made with the cheaper off-cuts of smoked salmon. The additional ingredients – mushrooms, tomatoes and chopped green pepper – add colour and texture to a classic dish.

6 medium eggs
50g (2oz) smoked salmon, chopped
50g (2oz) button mushrooms, chopped
3 small tomatoes, chopped
½ medium green pepper, de-seeded, cut into strips and chopped
12g (½oz) low-fat spread
6tbsps (90ml) semi-skimmed milk
black pepper to taste
1tbsp (15ml) fresh dill or parsley to garnish

1. Beat eggs in a bowl and mix in chopped smoked salmon, mushrooms, tomatoes and green pepper.
2. Heat low-fat spread and milk in a non-stick pan and add egg mixture. Season and scramble until creamy, using a fork.
3. Serve garnished with chopped dill or parsley, with crispbreads or a slice of wholemeal toast, cut into triangles.

Serves: 4
Per portion: Calories 183, Protein 16g, Fat 12g, Carbohydrate 3g, Fibre 1g.

Saucy Beans on Toast (v)

Soy sauce gives this favourite a new, tangy flavour. Children will love this for breakfast and as a teatime snack. Serve it with 'free' extras like mushrooms, tomatoes or sliced cucumber if you like, washed down with some chilled orange juice.

1 large onion, peeled and finely sliced
1tbsp (15ml) olive oil
1tbsp (15ml) English mustard
1tbsp (15ml) wine vinegar
2tbsp light soy sauce
1tbsp (15ml) Worcestershire Sauce
425g can baked beans
freshly ground black pepper to taste
4 slices wholemeal toast

1. Cook onion gently in the oil until soft. Add mustard, vinegar and sauces. Bring to the boil, add beans and reheat. Season with black pepper.

2. Toast bread and serve beans on top.

Serves: 4
Per portion: Calories 207, Protein 10g, Fat 6g, Carbohydrate 34g. Fibre 6g.

Light Meals

The two big advantages of taking a packed lunch to work are that you save cash and can control what you eat. Here are six lunch ideas which are easy to prepare. Five of them can be packed in a plastic container. The jacket potato toppings can be added to any 200g potato – so if you have a microwave oven at work, it's easy to whip up a tasty filling potato meal in about 10 minutes. Add 'free' salad, fresh fruit and one of your Carbohydrate Boosters™ for a satisfying feast that won't cost a mint.

Apple and Kipper Salad

Boil-in-the-bag kipper fillets can be used for this delicious salad, cutting down on preparation time. Add a squeeze of lemon and a dash of freshly ground black pepper. Lovely!

350g (14 oz) boil-in-the-bag kipper fillets
50g (2oz) long-grain brown rice
3tbsps (3 x 15ml) lemon juice
3tbsps (3 x 15ml) chopped fresh parsley and coriander
2 medium red eating apples, cored and chopped into
small pieces

1. Poach kipper fillets according to instructions, remove from bag and flake into a bowl. Be careful to remove all skin and bones.
2. Cook rice in plenty of boiling water for about 20 minutes, until tender. Strain.
3. Combine rice with kipper, lemon juice, parsley, coriander and chopped apple.

Serves: 2
Per portion: Calories 273, Protein 27g, Fat 12g, Carbohydrate 16g, Fibre 1g.

Greek Tzatsiki (v)

This is one of the easiest Greek specialities to make, and is absolutely delicious with wholemeal pitta bread and 'free' salad items such as grated carrot, raw mushrooms and beansprouts. It is also a cool, tasty side-dish to serve with curry.

1 cucumber, peeled
275ml (½pt) natural low-fat yogurt
2tbsps (2 x 15ml) lemon juice
2tbsps (2 x 15ml) chopped fresh spring onions
(include green part)
2tbsps (2 x 15ml) chopped fresh parsley
2 garlic cloves, peeled and crushed (optional)
freshly ground black pepper and a little salt to taste

1. Chop cucumber finely and mix together with all the other ingredients in a bowl.
2. Pack in a covered plastic dish with a well-fitting lid to transport safely.

Serves: 2
Per portion: Calories 51, Protein 4.5g, Fat 1g, Carbohydrate 7g, Fibre neg

Tomato, Cauliflower and Tarragon Soup (v)

Home-made soups are easy to carry in a wide-necked vacuum flask. You can make this soup with any of the 'free' vegetables on page 56, but tomato and cauliflower go very well together, especially when combined with tarragon and sherry!

1tbsp (15ml) olive oil
1 medium onion, peeled and chopped
3tbsps (45ml) cooking sherry
225g (8oz) cauliflower, cut into florets
225g (8oz) tomatoes, skinned and roughly chopped
750ml (1¼pt) vegetable stock
½tsp (2.5ml) sugar
1tsp (5ml) dried or 1tbsp (15ml) freshly chopped
tarragon (reserve a little for garnish)
a little salt and freshly ground black pepper to taste

1. Cook onion gently in the oil until soft. Add cooking sherry and bring to the boil.
2. Add cauliflower, tomatoes, vegetable stock, sugar, tarragon and seasoning. Bring to the boil and simmer for 45 mintues.
3. Liquidise or rub through a sieve. Correct seasoning and consistency (add a little more stock if necessary), reheat and serve sprinkled with a little more tarragon.

Serves: 2
Per portion: Calories 142, Protein 5g, Fat 9g, Carbohydrate 11g, Fibre 3.5g.

Pasta Salad (v)

Pasta is always satisfying, and it is very easy to eat at your desk with a spoon or fork. You can even work at the same time! This basic recipe can be used with additional chopped vegetables from your 'free' list or a tablespoon of sweetcorn. it is Carb loaded.

100g (4oz) wholemeal pasta twists or shells
2tbsps (2 x 15ml) fat-free salad dressing
1tbsp (15ml) wine vinegar
2tbsps (2 x 15ml) tomato paste
½tsp (2.5ml) dried oregano
salt and freshly ground black pepper
½ onion, peeled and finely chopped
3 sticks celery, finely chopped
½ red or green pepper, de-seeded and chopped
4tbsps (4 x 15ml) frozen or fresh peas, cooked
50g (2oz) Edam cheese, cubed
1tbsp (15ml) chopped fresh parsley

1. Cook pasta in boiling salted water, until just tender. Mix salad dressing, vinegar, tomato paste, oregano and seasoning.
2. Drain pasta, pour tomato dressing over the top. Leave to cool. Add onion, celery, red or green pepper, peas and cubes of cheese. Garnish with chopped parsley.

Serves: 4
Per portion: Calories 301, Protein 15g, Fat 8g, Carbohydrate 45g, Fibre 4.5g.

Cheese Terrine (v)

This well-flavoured terrine is delicious for lunch, served with some crusty bread and a mug of soup. Or, you could dish it up for a dinner party, garnished with slices of cucumber. It is suitable for vegetarians if vegetable instead of beef stock is used.

150g (6oz) lentils, soaked overnight
1 garlic clove, peeled and crushed
1 small onion, peeled and finely chopped
1 green pepper, de-seeded and chopped
50g (2oz) Red Leicester cheese, grated
2tbsps (2 x 15ml) chopped fresh parsley
2 medium eggs, beaten
3tbsps (3 x 15ml) beef or vegetable stock
1tsp (5ml) French mustard
salt and freshly ground black pepper
watercress to garnish

1. Drain lentils, place in a pan with water to cover, add crushed garlic and bring to the boil. Simmer for 2 minutes or until tender. Drain thoroughly.
2. Mix lentils with onion, pepper, cheese, parsley, beaten eggs, stock, mustard, salt and pepper.
3. Put mixture into a greased and lined 400g (1lb) loaf tin. Cover with lightly greased foil and bake in a preheated oven at 350°F, 180°C, Gas Mark 4, for 1 hr. Allow to cool, turn out and serve in slices. Garnish with watercress.

Serves: 4
Per portion: Calories 231, Protein 16g, Fat 8g, Carbohydrate 24.5g, Fibre 2.5g.

Jacket Potato Toppings

Here are six unusual ideas for lunchtime jacket potato toppings.
Cook a 200g (7oz) potato, remove from the oven, cut a thin
horizontal slice from the top, fluff up the centre and top with
one of these ideas:

1. Pesto Passion (v): add 1tsp (5ml) pesto sauce to 12g (1½oz)
low-fat spread and spoon on top of the potato. Delicious served
with cooked chopped spinach.

Serves: 1
Per portion: Calories 68, Protein 1g, Fat 7g, Carbohydrate neg,
Fibre 0.1g.

2. Yogurt Tingler (v): top potato with 2tbsps (2 x 15ml) natural
low-fat yogurt, and 1tsp (5ml) of hot Salsa sauce – the fiery taste is
luscious with the coolness of the yogurt.

Serves: 1
Per portion: Calories 20, Protein 2g, Fat neg, Carbohydrate 3g,
Fibre 2g.

3. Cheese and Mango Munch (v): mix 1tbsp (15ml) sweet
mango chutney with 12g (½oz) grated cheese or chopped soft
cheese (e.g. Camembert or Brie).

Serves: 1
Per portion: Calories 69, Protein 3g, Fat 4g,
Carbohydrate 5g, Fibre neg.

4. Seafood Surprise: Mix 25g (1oz) shelled, cooked prawns with 2tbsps (2 x 15ml) Crosse & Blackwell Waistline Low Fat Cocktail dressing and top with 1tbsp (15ml) fromage frais, 1tsp (5ml) lemon juice, freshly ground black pepper and garnish with chopped fresh parsley.

Serves: 1
Per portion: Calories 80, Protein 7g, Fat 3g, Carbohydrate 5g, Fibre neg.

5. Tomatoes and Basil (v): Heat 1 large, ripe tomato, chopped, or 1 small can of chopped Italian tomatoes, mix with 1tbsp (15ml) chopped fresh basil and pour over potato. Top with ½tsp (2.5ml) Parmesan cheese for extra Italian flavour.

Serves: 1
Per portion: Calories 128, Protein 1g, Fat neg, Carbohydrate 2g, Fibre 0.5g.

6. Curry Treat (v): Mix 1tsp (1 x 5ml) curry powder with 2tsps (2 x 5ml) mango chutney, 1tbsp (15ml) low-fat fromage frais and 1tbsp (15ml) sultanas. Pour over potato.

Serves: 1
Per portion: Calories 87, Protein 1g, Fat 2g, Carbohydrate 16g, Fibre 1g.

Main Meals

Starters

Melon with Prawns and Mango

This is an elegant starter for a dinner party, but would also be delicious piled on top of salad leaves for lunch.

1 ripe melon, well chilled
100g (4oz) shelled, cooked prawns
150ml (¼pt) low-fat fromage frais
2tsps (2 x 5ml) sweet mango chutney
pinch of salt and curry powder
sprigs of fresh mint to garnish

1. Halve the melon, discard seeds and scoop out melon balls with a small teaspoon or melon baller. Place in a dish with the prawns and keep chilled.
2. Just before serving, mix together the fromage frais and mango chutney, season with salt and a little curry powder. Divide the melon and prawns into four individual glass dishes and pour a little of the sauce over each. Decorate with mint sprigs.

Serves: 4
Per portion: Calories 93, Protein 9.5g, Fat 0.5g, Carbohydrate 14g, Fibre 1g.

Teriyaki Chicken

This makes an unusual starter, or it can be served as 'finger food' for a party, if allowed to cool slightly before serving. Make sure your guests have paper napkins to hold these delicious nibbles.

2 boned chicken breasts (200–300g/7–10oz)
2tsps (2 x 5ml) vegetable oil
120ml (4fl oz) dry white wine or sake
120ml (4fl oz) medium sweet sherry
60ml (2fl oz) soy sauce
1tbsp (15ml) sugar
2 cloves garlic, peeled and crushed
lemon wedges, coriander sprigs and cucumber slices
to garnish

1. Heat the oil in a shallow pan and brown the chicken pieces. Remove chicken and reserve.

2. Combine the remaining ingredients in a dish, pour into the pan and bring to the boil. Replace the chicken and cook gently, turning the chicken repeatedly, until the sauce is reduced and the chicken is thickly coated – approximately 10 minutes.

3. Remove chicken, place on a board and cut into 5cm (2 in) pieces. Place on a warmed dish and garnish with lemon, coriander and cucumber.

Serves: 4
Per portion: Calories 105, Protein 0.5g, Fat 2.7g, Carbohydrate 8.4g, Fibre 0.

Borsch

A delicious starter for a winter evening, or serve the soup for lunch with a hunk of crusty wholemeal bread and fruit to follow.

400g (1lb) onions, peeled and finely chopped
2tbsps (2 x 15ml) olive oil
1 clove garlic, peeled and finely chopped
3tbsps (3 x 15ml) dark brown sugar
600g (1½lb) raw beetroot, peeled and coarsely grated
(long-life, pre-cooked, vacuum-packed beetroot is also
available)
6tbsps (6 x 15ml) balsamic vinegar
900ml (1½pt) chicken stock
150ml (¼pt) natural low-fat yogurt
chopped fresh parsley to garnish

1. Sauté the onion in the oil in a large saucepan until soft, but not coloured. Add the garlic and brown sugar and cook gently for about 3 minutes, stirring all the time.
2. Add beetroot, vinegar, chicken stock and about 450ml (¾pt) water and bring to the boil. Simmer, stirring occasionally, for about 45 minutes (if raw) or until the beetroot is tender. Season to taste.
3. Ladle into four bowls and top each one with 1tbsp (1 x 15ml) of yogurt and a sprinkling of chopped parsley.

Serves: 4
Per portion: Calories 172, Protein 6.7g, Fat 0.7g,
Carbohydrate 37g, Fibre 4.3g.

Onions in White Wine (v)

This dish is scrumptious served cold. Serve it alone or as part of a cold hors d'oeuvres selection which could include ratatouille, tomato salad and perhaps some cold baked fish such as salmon, tuna or salt cod.

800g (2lb) small onions, placed in warm water
to soften skins before peeling
600ml (1pt) water
300ml (½pt) dry white wine
125g (5oz) sugar
125g (5oz) raisins (pre-soaked in water
for 10 minutes to plump up)
4tbsps (4 x 15ml) tomato purée
3tbsps (3 x 15ml) olive oil
4tbsps (4 x 15ml) white wine vinegar
salt and freshly ground black pepper
a sprinkling of cayenne pepper to taste
chopped fresh parsley to garnish

1. Place onions in a large saucepan with the water, dry white wine, sugar, raisins, tomato purée and olive oil.
2. Add the wine vinegar and seasoning to taste. Bring to the boil and simmer gently for about 45 minutes until onions are tender, but still retain their shape.
3. Remove the onions from the sauce and arrange in a serving dish.
4. Place the sauce back on the hob and turn up the heat. Allow the sauce to boil and reduce by half to thicken and concentrate the flavours. Pour over the onions and raisins.
5. Chill and serve cold, garnished with chopped fresh parsley.

Serves: 4
Per portion: Calories 445, Protein 4g, Fat 12g,
Carbohydrate 73g, Fibre 4g.

Raspberry and Kiwi Appetiser (v)

This starter could easily be served as a pudding instead – just add some fromage frais or Greek yogurt. However, the lime juice makes it a very refreshing appetiser indeed, especially on a warm evening.

200g (7oz) raspberries
2tbsps (2 x 15ml) sugar
1 ripe Williams pear
juice of ½ lemon and 1 lime
2 canned peach halves
4 canned apricot halves
3tbsps (3 x 15ml) canned drained mandarin segments
(all fruit in this recipe should be canned in natural juice, not syrup)
2 kiwi fruit
sprigs of fresh mint leaves to garnish

1. Place the raspberries in a large bowl with the sugar.
2. Peel, quarter and core the pear, cut into thin wedges and place on a dish. Sprinkle with the lemon juice and leave for 5 minutes.
3. Drain peach and apricot halves and slice. Drain mandarin segments.
4. Mix the pear, peach and apricot slices and mandarin segments with the raspberries and lime juice.
5. Thinly peel and slice the kiwi fruit, and arrange in a ring on four individual dishes. Pile the fruit mixture on top and garnish with fresh mint leaves.

Serves: 4
Per portion: Calories 82, Protein 1g, Fat neg,
Carbohydrate 19.6g, Fibre 2.8g.

Oriental Kebabs

These cook well on a barbecue as well as under a conventional grill. The marinade can be made the day before. This makes an ideal starter for hungry guests or double up the quantities and serve with rice and a huge salad as a main course.

2tbsps (2 x 15ml) soy sauce
5tbsps (5 x 15ml) clear honey
1tsp (5ml) ground ginger
juice of ½ lemon
400g (1lb) pork fillet, cut into 3cm (1in) cubes
1 large green and 1 large red pepper, de-seeded
and cut into cubes
4 small onions, peeled and halved
2 apples, quartered and cored
8 medium closed-cup mushrooms
freshly ground pepper and a little salt to taste
1 lemon, sliced to garnish
4 spring onions to garnish

1. In a large bowl, mix together the soy sauce, honey, ground ginger and lemon juice. Add pork and leave to marinate for 4 hours, or overnight.
2. Thread meat on to four skewers, alternating with pieces of pepper, onion, apple and mushrooms.
3. Season with plenty of freshly ground pepper and a little salt. Place under a hot grill, turning often until the meat is cooked through (approximately 10 minutes), and basting with the remaining marinade. Garnish with slices of lemon and spring onion 'tassels'.

Serves: 4
Per portion: Calories 294, Protein 36g, Fat 4g, Carbohydrate 29g, Fibre 3g.

Main Courses

Economical family dishes that are quick to cook, and will be enjoyed by slimmers and non-slimmers alike.

Turkey with Apricots and Ginger

This is very simple, but absolutely delicious. Serve with a huge salad and a little brown rice to soak up the scrumptious sauce.

100g (4oz) dried apricots
1tsp (5ml) ground ginger
1tsp (5ml) sugar
4 x 100–125g (approx 4oz each) turkey fillets
150ml (¼pt) dry white wine
fresh coriander sprigs to garnish

1. Place the apricots in a bowl, just cover with water and add the ground ginger and sugar. Leave to stand overnight.
2. Place the turkey fillets on the grid of a grill pan and spoon over a little of the apricot liquid. Cook under a hot grill for about 10 minutes, turning once.
3. Meanwhile, simmer the apricots and the rest of the liquid for about 10 minutes, then liquidise to a smooth sauce in a blender.
4. Place the cooked fillets on to a heated serving dish and keep warm. Pour the turkey juices from the grill pan into a saucepan and add the white wine. Place the pan on to the heat and allow mixture to boil until reduced by half. Add the apricot and ginger sauce to the saucepan and mix well with the reduced wine, stirring all the time until boiling point is reached.
5. Pour the sauce over the turkey fillets and garnish with sprigs of fresh coriander.

Serves: 4
Per portion: Calories 205, Protein 35.5g, Fat 2g, Carbohydrate 6g, Fibre neg.

Boston Baked Beans (v)

Once you've tasted these, you'll never want to open another can!
Seriously, they are delicious and with hunks of crusty bread, they'll
fill up a hungry family. Good for lunch, supper and suitable for
vegetarians.

400g (1lb) dried haricot beans, soaked in water overnight
2 medium onions, peeled and finely chopped
400g (1lb) tomatoes, skinned and chopped
3tbsps (3 x 15ml) molasses
2tsps (2 x 5ml) raw brown sugar
2tsps (2 x 15ml) mustard powder
1tsp (15ml) chopped fresh herbs such as sage, thyme,
rosemary or parsley
2tbsps (2 x 15ml) tomato purée
2tbsps (2 x 15ml) Worcestershire Sauce
salt to taste and plenty of freshly ground black pepper

1. Drain beans and cook in plenty of fresh water for about
40 minutes, until almost tender. Add more water if necessary,
while the beans are cooking, so they are always covered.
2. Preheat oven to 325°F, 170°C, Gas Mark 3. Pour beans and
cooking liquor into an oven-proof casserole dish with a lid and add
the onion, tomato, molasses, sugar, mustard, herbs, tomato purée,
Worcestershire sauce, salt and freshly ground black pepper to
taste. Stir well and cover.
3. Bake for 3 hours, stirring occasionally, until the beans are tender.
If they seem a little dry during baking, add extra water. Adjust the
seasoning to taste and serve.

Serves: 4–6
Per portion: Calories 192, Protein 9.5g, Fat 1g,
Carbohydrate 36g, Fibre 9g.

Lemon Chicken

This makes a change from the usual roast chicken dishes and is a very economical dish when the family come to Sunday lunch. You can double up the quantities for a bigger crowd.

1 x 1.3kg (3–3½lb) oven-ready chicken, without giblets
2 small turnips, peeled and cut into large chunks
2 small carrots, peeled and cut into large chunks
1 lemon, juice and grated rind
1 medium onion, peeled and roughly chopped
2tsps (2 x 5ml) white wine vinegar
salt and freshly ground black pepper
50g (2oz) sugar
1tbsp (1 x 15ml) cornflour
slices of lemon and sprigs of parsley to garnish

1. Put the chicken into a large saucepan with the turnips, carrots, lemon rind, onion, white wine vinegar and a little salt and pepper. Cover with water and bring to the boil, then cover with a lid and simmer for about 1–1½ hours. To check if the chicken is cooked, test with a skewer in the thickest part of the thigh. The skewer should penetrate without pressure and the juices released should run clear.
2. Remove the chicken from the pan. Spoon 300ml (½pt) of the liquid into another saucepan with the lemon juice, white wine vinegar and sugar. Simmer for about 3 minutes.
3. Blend the cornflour with a little of the remaining liquid. Add to the lemon juice mixture and cook for 3 minutes until the sauce is fairly thick and almost transparent.
4. Carve the chicken into slices, place on a heated serving dish and pour over the sauce. Garnish with slices of lemon and chopped parsley.

Serves: 4
Per portion: Calories 272, Protein 30g, Fat 8g, Carbohydrate 22.5g, Fibre 2g.

Piquant Fish Casserole

This is very simple to cook for a midweek supper, and you can use any kind of fresh or frozen white fish – cod, coley or even a more expensive fish like haddock or turbot if you are feeling flush!

4 x 100–125g (approx 4oz) pieces of white fish
juice of 1 lemon
30ml (1fl oz) water
2tsps (2 x 5ml) Worcestershire Sauce
1tsp (5ml) French mustard
1tsp (5ml) sugar
salt and freshly ground black pepper to taste
parsley sprigs and lemon wedges to garnish

1. Place the fish in a shallow casserole dish. Mix together the remaining ingredients and pour on top.
2. Cover and cook in a preheated oven at 375°F, 190°C, Gas Mark 5, for about 20 minutes or until fish is cooked. Serve garnished with lemon wedges and parsley sprigs.

Serves: 4
Per portion: Calories 143, Protein 21g, Fat 5g, Carbohydrate 3g, Fibre 0.

Oodles of Noodles Stir-Fry

This is incredibly quick to whizz up in a wok or large frying pan and tastes wonderful. It is also very filling and there is lots of it because the noodles are so light. You can use any leftover lean cooked meat and most supermarkets now sell water chestnuts and beansprouts.

1tbsp (15ml) corn oil
1tbsp (15ml) sesame oil
50g (2oz) onion, peeled and chopped
3cm (1in) piece fresh ginger, peeled and chopped
50g (2oz) red pepper, de-seeded and sliced
50g (2oz) fresh broccoli cut into small florets
50g (2oz) water chestnuts
50g (2oz) beansprouts
100g (4oz) lean cooked meat or poultry (no skin)
100g (4oz) peeled prawns
2tbsps (2 x 15ml) light soy sauce
1tsp (5ml) sugar
150g (5oz) thin Chinese noodles
4 spring onion tassels to garnish

1. Heat both oils in a wok or large, non-stick frying pan. Stir-fry the chopped onion, ginger and pepper for 1 minute.
2. Add the broccoli, water chestnuts and beansprouts and stir-fry for about 2 minutes. Add the meat and prawns and heat through.
3. Mix the soy sauce with the sugar and add to the pan. Meanwhile, cook the noodles in boiling salted water for about 5 minutes.
4. Drain well, add to the stir-fry and toss through the meat, prawns and vegetables until everything is mixed. Pile on to a heated plate and serve garnished with spring onion tassels.

Serves: 4
Per portion: Calories 192, Protein 18g, Fat 9g, Carbohydrate 11g, Fibre 1g.

ITALIAN

Italian dishes always seem to taste of pure sunshine! These are some favourites, given a new twist for System S.

Mozzarella and Tomato Salad (v)

A light, oil-free dressing saves calories on this classic Italian starter. Add prawns or cooked chicken if you want to turn it into a main course salad dish.

4 large beef tomatoes
150g (6oz) Italian mozzarella cheese
5tbsp (5 x 15ml) oil-free dressing
1 clove garlic, peeled and crushed
2tsps (2 x 5ml) lemon juice
1tsp (5ml) sugar
salt and freshly ground black pepper
fresh basil leaves to garnish

1. Slice the tomatoes horizontally, and the cheese very finely.
2. Arrange alternate, overlapping slices of tomato and cheese on four plates. Mix the oil-free dressing, garlic, lemon juice, sugar and seasoning together and spoon over the dish. Garnish with chopped basil leaves.

Serves: 4
Per portion: Calories 140, Protein 10.5g, Fat 8g, Carbohydrate 6g, Fibre 1.5g.

Spinach Lasagne

600ml (1pt) skimmed milk
50g (2oz) flour
25g (1oz) margarine
1 400g can chopped tomatoes
1 375g can ratatouille
250g frozen spinach, cooked and drained
¼tsp ground mace
1tsp mixed herbs
1tsp dried basil
325g (12oz) lasagne (non pre-cook)
150g (5oz) mushrooms, sliced
100g (4oz) Cheddar cheese, finely grated

1. Place milk, flour and margarine into a pan. Place over heat and whisk continuously until sauce begins to thicken (a balloon whisk works well).

2. Mix together tomatoes, ratatouille and spinach in a bowl. Add the mace, mixed herbs and basil. Mix again.

3. Put a layer of lasagne to cover the bottom of a 20 x 30cm (8 x 12in) dish. Pour in half the tomato mixture and then cover with another layer of lasagne.

4. Pour in half the white sauce and all the mushrooms and cover with a layer of lasagne, followed by the remainder of the tomato mixture.

5. Finish with a final layer of lasagne and the remainder of the white sauce. Sprinkle with cheese.

6. Bake for 40–45 minutes in a preheated oven at 350°F, 180°C, Gas Mark 4.

Serves: 6
Per portion: Calories 340, Protein 13g, Fat 10g, Carbohydrate 54g, Fibre 5g.

Bruschetta with Tomatoes (v)

This is a classic Italian dish which is delicious served for lunch or Saturday brunch with friends.

4 slices crusty white Italian bread
1 clove garlic
2tbsps (2 x 15ml) oil-free dressing
1tsp (5ml) sugar
4 large, ripe tomatoes, roughly chopped
salt and freshly ground black pepper
fresh basil leaves to garnish

1. Toast the bread on both sides under a hot grill. Cut the garlic clove in half and rub it over one side of the toasted bread.
2. Mix together the oil-free dressing and sugar and dribble over the bread. Spoon the tomatoes over, season and garnish with the basil. Eat while the toast is still hot.

Serves: 4
Per portion: Calories 292, Protein 10g, Fat 3g,
Carbohydrate 60g, Fibre 2g.

Spaghettini
with Prawns and Garlic

Spaghettini, which is much finer than spaghetti, is particularly good with seafood. This recipe includes chilli powder to add a kick to the basic sauce.

200g (8oz) spaghettini or angel hair spaghetti
1dsp (10ml) olive oil
100g (4oz) onion, peeled and finely chopped
2 cloves garlic, peeled and crushed
½tsp (2.5ml) chilli powder (or to taste)
400g can chopped tomatoes
500g (17oz) passata (sieved tomatoes)
300g (11oz) peeled prawns
salt and freshly ground black pepper
2tsps (2 x 5ml) sugar
4 whole prawns and finely chopped fresh parsley
or dill to garnish

1. Cook spaghettini in plenty of boiling water until 'al dente' or firm, yet tender.
2. Heat the oil in a large pan and stir-fry the onion, garlic and chilli powder. Add tomatoes and passata and simmer for about 20 minutes.
3. Stir in prawns, cook for 2–3 minutes, season to taste and add sugar.
4. Drain pasta, pile into a heated bowl, pour on the sauce and garnish with prawns and parsley or dill.

Serves: 4
Per portion: Calories 321, Protein 25g, Fat 5g, Carbohydrate 48g, Fibre 3g.

ORIENTAL (THAI, CHINESE, INDIAN)

The delicate flavours, exotic ingredients and sensual textures of oriental food are perfect for slimmers. These six recipes prove that you don't need to eat bland dishes to lose weight!

Thai Baked Trout

This is so tasty, you'll wonder why you ever served trout with boring old almonds! As in most Thai dishes, there are a lot of ingredients. However, most of the work is in chopping them up – the actual cooking is easy. Just make sure you don't overbake the trout.

4 medium trout, cleaned and gutted, but with the heads left on
salt and freshly ground black pepper

Stuffing:
5cm (2in) piece of root ginger, peeled and finely chopped
4 spring onions, chopped
50g (2oz) back bacon, grilled, de-rinded and finely chopped
50g (2oz) canned bamboo shoots, drained and shredded
2tbsps (2 x 15ml) chopped fresh coriander leaves
juice and grated zest of 2 lemons and 2 limes

Sauce:
1tbsp (15ml) cornflour
2tbsps (2 x 15ml) water
150ml (¼pt) fish stock or water
2tbsps (2 x 15ml) each of light soy sauce, soft brown sugar, dry sherry and tomato purée
2tbsps (2 x 15ml) sweet chilli sauce

1. Preheat the oven to 375°F, 190°C, Gas Mark 5. Mix together the ginger, spring onions, bacon, bamboo shoots, coriander (reserving some to garnish) and lemon and lime zest. Divide mixture into four portions and stuff inside the fish.

2. Place the fish, head to tail, in a shallow oven-proof dish, squeeze over the lemon and lime juices, season and cover with lightly oiled foil. Bake the trout in the oven for approximately 25 minutes.

3. Meanwhile, blend the cornflour with the water in a small pan. Add the rest of the sauce ingredients, bring to the boil and simmer, stirring all the time, for 2 minutes. When the fish is cooked, pour off the cooking juice into the pan and blend with the sauce.

4. Pour sauce over the fish and serve garnished with coriander.

Serves: 4

Per portion: Calories 252, Protein 33g, Fat 11g, Carbohydrate 6g, Fibre 0.5g.

Chinese Lamb

This is a very filling main course dish, especially if served with rice or Chinese noodles as an accompaniment. It's best to use a wok, but a non-stick frying pan will do.

1tbsp (15ml) oil
400g (1lb) lean lamb, thinly sliced
200g (7oz) carrots, sliced diagonally or in
thick matchsticks
4 celery sticks, sliced diagonally
3tbsps (3 x 15ml) soy sauce
4tbsps (4 x 15ml) dry sherry
2 leeks, sliced diagonally
4 cloves garlic, peeled and thinly sliced
100g (4oz) mange-tout, cut in half diagonally
4 spring onions, chopped

5cm (2in) piece root ginger, peeled and finely chopped
1tsp (5ml) crushed black peppercorns
2tsps (2 x 5ml) sugar
lemon or lime slices and fresh coriander leaves to
garnish

1. Heat the oil in a wok or deep frying pan. Add the lamb and
brown on both sides.

2. Lower the heat, add the carrots and celery and stir-fry for 3
minutes. Add the soy sauce and sherry. Stir and cover, cooking for
between 5 and 10 minutes. The vegetables should be tender, but
still have 'bite' appeal.

3. Add leeks, garlic, mange-tout, spring onions and ginger and
cook for 1 minute. Add peppercorns and sugar. Heat through.

4. Serve in the wok or on a heated dish, garnished with lemon or
lime slices and coriander leaves.

Serves: 4
Per portion: Calories 306, Protein 22g, Fat 18g,
Carbohydrate 11g, Fibre 3g.

Stir-Fried Tofu and Vegetables (v)

This makes a quick supper dish and is suitable for vegetarians. Tofu
is excellent for stir-frying, as it absorbs the flavours of the different
ingredients, including garlic, chilli paste and mushrooms. Non-
vegetarians can add shredded pork or a few prawns to this recipe.

2 x 285g (2 x 10oz) cakes of tofu (each one is enough
for 2 people)
2tbsps (2 x 15ml) vegetable oil
1 clove garlic, peeled and sliced
2 small leeks, sliced diagonally
2 celery sticks, sliced diagonally

150g (5oz) button mushrooms, sliced
150g (5oz) small broccoli florets
4 dried chillies, left whole
1tbsp (15ml) chilli paste
1tbsp (15ml) dry sherry
2tsps (2 x 5ml) sugar
1 lime, cut into wedges to garnish
1tbsp (1 x 15ml) chopped coriander or spring onions
to garnish

1. Cut each piece of tofu into 8 pieces.

2. Heat a little oil in a wok or non-stick frying pan, add the garlic, leeks and celery and stir-fry for 1 minute. Stir in the mushrooms and broccoli and cook for 2 minutes. Remove this mixture from the pan with a slotted spoon and set aside, ensuring it remains hot.

3. Add a little more oil if necessary, add the tofu and fry for 2 minutes. Drain on kitchen paper. Return the vegetables and the tofu to the wok, stir in the chillies, chilli paste, sherry and sugar and cook for 1 minute.

4. Remove the dried chillies and serve straight from the pan, garnished with lime wedges and coriander or spring onion.

Serves: 4
Per portion: Calories 211, Protein 14g, Fat 14g, Carbohydrate 6g, Fibre 2g.

Cantonese Beef

This is a delicious, quickie meal for a dinner party or Sunday lunch. You can buy oyster sauce in most supermarkets nowadays and dry sherry makes a good substitute for Chinese rice wine. The beef is so tender that it almost melts in your mouth.

250–350g (9–12oz) lean beef (use sirloin, rump or
other tender cut), cut into thin slices

**1tsp (1 x 5ml) each salt, sugar, soy sauce, Chinese
rice wine or dry sherry, cornflour
1 head Chinese leaves or cos lettuce, shredded
2tbsps (2 x 15ml) olive oil
1 spring onion, finely chopped
1.25cm (½in) root ginger, peeled and finely chopped
1tbsp (15ml) oyster sauce**

1. Place beef in a bowl with pinch of salt, the sugar, soy sauce, rice
wine or sherry and cornflour. Mix together and leave to marinate for
1 hour.
2. Wash the Chinese leaves or lettuce, and cut each leaf into two
or three pieces.
3. Heat a little oil in a hot wok until smoking, add the Chinese
leaves or lettuce and stir-fry lightly for 1 minute. Remove with a
slotted spoon and arrange on a warmed serving dish.
4. Now add a little more oil if necessary, add the spring onion and
ginger, then the beef and marinade. When the beef starts changing
colour, add the oyster sauce and stir-fry for 1 minute. Serve on the
Chinese leaves or lettuce.

Serves: 3
Per portion: Calories 287, Protein 26g, Fat 18g,
Carbohydrate 7g, Fibre 2g.

Mussels with
Lime and Lemon Grass

You can buy fresh or vacuum-sealed mussels in most
supermarkets. They make a tasty, inexpensive supper dish,
especially when given a special 'kick' with this Thai-style sauce.

Serve with a wedge of crusty wholemeal bread (which adds about 100 calories per portion to the recipe calorie total).

750g (1¾lb) live mussels
3 shallots, peeled and finely chopped
2 cloves garlic, peeled and finely chopped
300ml (½pt) hot vegetable stock
1 stalk lemon grass
2 Kaffir lime leaves
2tbsps (2 x 15ml) chopped fresh coriander
finely grated rind and juice of 2 limes and 2 lemons
2tsps (2 x 5ml) sugar
1 lime cut into wedges and fresh coriander leaves
to garnish

1. Wash mussels under cold running water, using a sharp knife to scrape off the beards. Discard any that are damaged or remain open when tapped. Rinse well with several changes of water.
2. Place the chopped shallots and garlic in a large pan with a little of the vegetable stock and cook for 2–3 minutes until softened.
3. Bruise the lemon grass with a rolling pin and add to the pan with the lime leaves, coriander, grated lemon and lime rind and juice, sugar, mussels and the rest of the stock. Put the lid on the pan and cook for 3–5 minutes over moderate heat, shaking the saucepan from time to time.
4. Check that all the mussels have opened (discard any that have not), lift them out on to two plates, reduce the remaining liquid slightly by boiling rapidly, remove lemon grass and lime leaves and pour over the mussels.
5. Garnish with lime wedges and coriander leaves.

Serves: 2
Per portion: Calories 317, Protein 47g, Fat 7.5g, Carbohydrate 17g, Fibre 1g.

Spicy Vegetable Curry (v)

You can make this in quantity and freeze it. The fabulous flavours seem to mature during freezing. It is delicious, served for lunch with an exotic passion fruit yogurt to follow. Vary the vegetables according to season and availability.

1tsp (5ml) fennel seeds
2 onions, peeled and sliced
400g can chopped tomatoes
150ml (¼pt) passata
1tsp (5ml) each ground coriander, ground cumin and
chilli powder
2tsps (2 x 5ml) root ginger, peeled and finely chopped
2tsps (2 x 5ml) sugar
2 cloves garlic, peeled and crushed
1 small aubergine, thinly sliced
1 medium potato, peeled and cubed
1 green pepper, de-seeded and finely chopped
3 courgettes, sliced
2 green chillies, de-seeded and finely chopped
salt
50g (2oz) frozen peas
4 slices fresh or canned pineapple (in juice) cut into
1.25 cm (½in) pieces

1. Place the fennel seeds and sliced onions in a pan and add the canned tomatoes and passata. Cook gently over a moderate heat until the onions are soft, about 3 minutes.
2. Lower the heat and add the coriander, cumin and chilli powder. Cook, stirring for 1 minute. Add the ginger, sugar, garlic, aubergine and potato, mix well and cook for about 15 minutes.
3. Add the green pepper, courgettes, chillies and a little salt to taste. Bring to the boil, then simmer for 10 minutes, stirring

occasionally and correcting the consistency by adding a little water
if necessary.

4. Stir in the peas and pineapple and cook for 3 minutes. Serve
immediately.

Serves: 4
Per portion: Calories 138, Protein 7g, Fat 1g,
Carbohydrate 27g, Fibre 5g.

SPANISH AND MEXICAN

There's been a terrific interest in Spanish and Mexican food
over the past few years. Some of the traditional dishes can
be high in fat, especially when ingredients are fried or soured
cream is added. This selection of dishes has all the taste, but
fat is kept to a minimum.

Cebiche

The fish in this traditional recipe is 'cooked' overnight in the lime and
orange juices. The fresher the fish, the better it tastes!

400g (1lb) cod or haddock fillets, skinned
1 medium onion, peeled and sliced finely
juice of 1 orange and 6 limes
1tbsp (15ml) olive oil
3tbsps (3 x 15ml) tomato ketchup
1tsp (5ml) each Worcestershire Sauce, dried oregano
and sugar
3 spring onions, peeled and sliced, to garnish

1. Cut the fish into bite-size pieces and remove any bones. Place in
a bowl with the onion and orange and lime juices. Stir so all the fish
is well covered.

2. Cover and leave in the refrigerator for at least 3 hours, or preferably overnight.

3. About an hour before serving, put the rest of the ingredients, except for the spring onions, into a bowl, stir well and pour over the fish. Stir gently, so the fish doesn't break. Serve cold, garnished with sliced spring onions.

Serves: 4
Per portion: Calories 149, Protein 19g, Fat 5g, Carbohydrate 8g, Fibre 1g.

Chilli Con Carne

There is no need to pre-fry the minced beef in oil for this recipe. If you simply brown it in a non-stick pan, you will save a lot of fat and calories. This is often served with rice, but it is also good with just a huge mixed salad and refreshing glass of chilled white wine.

400g (1lb) lean minced beef
1 small onion, peeled and finely chopped
1 garlic clove, peeled and crushed
300ml (½pt) beef stock
1tbsp (15ml) chilli powder (or to taste)
1tbsp (15ml) tomato purée
2tsps (2 x 5ml) sugar
6 ripe tomatoes, skinned, de-seeded and chopped
1 small red pepper, de-seeded and chopped
200g can kidney beans, drained and rinsed
4tbsps (4 x 15ml) natural low-fat yogurt and a
sprinkling of chilli powder to garnish

1. Place the beef in a non-stick frying pan and cook over moderate heat until browned. Drain off the fat.

2. Place the chopped onion and garlic clove in a large saucepan. Add a little of the beef stock, and cook gently until the onion is soft, about 3 minutes. Add the drained beef to the pan.

3. Stir in the chilli powder, cook for 1 minute, then add the tomato purée, sugar, remaining beef stock, red pepper and kidney beans. Cover and simmer gently for 20–25 minutes, until the minced beef is tender. Check and correct the consistency with additional water or stock and season to taste with salt and freshly ground black pepper.

4. Spoon on to four individual hot plates and garnish each one with a spoonful of yogurt and a sprinkling of chilli powder.

Serves: 4

Per portion: Calories 280, Protein 28g, Fat 11g, Carbohydrate 20g, Fibre 5g.

Marinated Pork Fillet

This is a low-fat version of the delicious pork served as a takeaway in many Mexican towns. You can serve it with warmed tortillas, plus a huge salad. It is also good threaded on to skewers and cooked over the barbecue.

Marinade:
1 medium onion, peeled and finely chopped
2 cloves garlic, peeled and crushed
1tsp (5ml) salt
½tsp (2.5ml) freshly ground black pepper
1tsp (5ml) sugar
4tbsps (4 x 15ml) malt vinegar
1.8kg (4lb) pork fillet or other lean pork cut into 5cm
(2in) pieces, fat removed
juice of 1 lemon
lemon wedges and chopped fresh parsley to garnish

1. Liquidise the marinade ingredients in a blender for 60 seconds at high speed. Smooth this paste all over the meat and leave for at least 2 hours or overnight.

2. Remove meat from marinade, place in a grill pan and cook under a hot grill, turning frequently. Towards the end of the cooking (about 15 minutes) pour over any remaining marinade and the lemon juice.

3. Serve hot, garnished with lemon wedges and chopped fresh parsley.

Serves: 8
Per portion: Calories 390, Protein 76g, Fat 9g, Carbohydrate 1g, Fibre neg

Tortilla Salad

This is a great salad for Mondays because you can use any cooked leftover meat or even cold cooked fish. The tortilla chips on top make it taste lovely and crunchy, and the chillies add a lot of 'bite' to the dressing.

1 cos or Webb's lettuce, finely shredded
½ onion, peeled and finely chopped
3 tomatoes, finely chopped
10 pitted black olives, finely sliced
2 green chillies, de-seeded and green flesh only, finely chopped
200g (7oz) cooked chicken, turkey, beef, prawns, tuna or other firm-textured fish (bones removed!), shredded
juice of 2 limes or small lemons
½tsp (2.5ml) salt
1tsp (5ml) sugar
freshly ground black pepper
1 small packet tortilla chips
coriander leaves and sliced spring onion to garnish

1. Mix together all the ingredients, except for the garnish, about 30 minutes before serving.

2. Top with tortilla chips, garnish with coriander and spring onions and serve.

Serves: 4
Per portion: Calories 228, Protein 20g, Fat 8g, Carbohydrate 20g, Fibre 4g.

Spanish Chicken

This is yummy served with tacos or tortillas, and makes a change from beef or lamb. If you prefer a milder taste, halve the quantity of green chillies.

2 large onions, peeled and thinly sliced
4 green peppers, de-seeded and cut into thin strips
4 green chillies, de-seeded and finely chopped
3tbsps (3 x 15ml) tomato purée
1 chicken stock cube
¼tsp (1.25ml) salt
freshly ground black pepper
1tsp (5ml) sugar
fresh coriander leaves
150ml (¼pt) water
100g (4oz) fat-reduced Cheddar cheese, grated
200g (7oz) cold roast chicken, skin removed, cut into chunks
150ml (¼pt) carton natural low-fat yogurt
fresh coriander leaves to garnish

1. Place the onion, peppers, chillies, tomato purée, crumbled stock cube, salt, pepper to taste, sugar and coriander in a pan. Add the water, stir and cover. Simmer gently for 15 minutes.
2. Stir in half of the cheese and the cooked chicken. Pour the

mixture into an oven-proof dish, stir in the yogurt and top with the rest of the grated cheese.

3. Bake for about 10 minutes in a preheated oven, at 350°F, 180°C, Gas Mark 4, until the cheese melts and turns golden brown. Garnish with coriander leaves.

Serves: 4
Per portion: Calories 242, Protein 31g, Fat 6g, Carbohydrate 17g, Fibre 4g.

Salad Dressings

Try these dressings to give your salads a fresh, fabulous taste without adding too many calories. All these recipes make enough dressing for four people.

Garlic and Yogurt (v)

Mix 3tbsps (3 x 15ml) reduced-calorie mayonnaise with 4tbsps (4 x 15ml) natural low-fat yogurt, 1 crushed clove garlic and 2 chopped spring onions.

Serves: 4
Per portion: Calories 42, Protein 1g, Fat 3g, Carbohydrate 2g, Fibre 0.5g.

Apple, Horseradish and Soft Cheese (v)

Mix 1tbsp (15ml) creamed horseradish sauce with 100g (4oz) Quark skimmed milk soft cheese, a little skimmed milk (2 x 15ml), 1 chopped apple, juice of 1 lemon and season with freshly ground black pepper.

Serves: 4
Per portion: Calories 38, Protein 4g, Fat 0.5g,
Carbohydrate 5g, Fibre 0.5g.

Oriental Ginger (v)

Mix 1tbsp (15ml) each light soy sauce, sesame oil and dry sherry
with ½tsp (2.5ml) Chinese five-spice powder, 1tsp (5ml) grated
fresh ginger, 1 crushed clove garlic and 1tsp (5ml) sugar.

Serves: 4
Per portion: Calories 85g, Protein 0.5g, Fat 7.5g,
Carbohydrate 2g, Fibre 0.

Tomato and Basil (v)

Mix 4tbsps (4 x 15ml) oil-free dressing with 2tbsps (2 x 15ml)
tomato juice, 1 crushed clove garlic, 1tbsp (15ml) fresh chopped
basil and salt and freshly ground black pepper to taste.

Serves: 4
Per portion: Calories 11, Protein neg, Fat neg,
Carbohydrate 2g, Fibre 0.

Hot Mexican (v)

Mix 2tbsps (2 x 15ml) enchillada sauce with 4tbsps (4 x 15ml) oil-
free French dressing, juice of 1 fresh lime, 1tsp (5ml) sugar and salt
and freshly ground black pepper to taste.

Serves: 4
Per portion: Calories 16, Protein neg, Fat neg,
Carbohydrate 4g, Fibre 0.

Dill and Lemon (v)

Mix 2tbsps (2 x 15ml) oil-free dressing, 3tbsps (3 x 15ml) lemon juice, 2 crushed cloves garlic, salt and freshly ground black pepper to taste, 1tsp (5ml) sugar and 1tbsp (15ml) fresh chopped dill.

Serves: 4
Per portion: Calories 12, Protein neg, Fat neg, Carbohydrate 3g, Fibre 0.

Perfect Puddings

These sweet treats are modest in calories and give you the carbohydrate boost you need to fight the fat!

Old-Fashioned Trifle (v)

This tastes wicked, but the aerosol dairy cream is light and low in calories, and the sherry adds so much flavour that it just has to be included.

6 trifle sponges
3tbsps (3 x 15ml) medium sweet sherry
1 packet raspberry jelly
215g (8oz) can fruit cocktail in water
1 packet instant custard

To decorate:
6 swirls aerosol cream, sprinkling of silver dragées,
hundreds and thousands or a little grated chocolate

1. Crumble the sponges and soak in the sherry. Place in the bottom of a glass bowl. Make up the jelly as instructed on the packet.

2. Pour it over the sponges and chill in the refrigerator until set. Top with the drained fruit. Make up the custard, let cool slightly, and spoon over the fruit. Chill again until set.

3. Serve topped with the aerosol cream and chosen decoration.

Serves: 4

Per portion: Calories 276, Protein 7g, Fat 10g, Carbohydrate 40g, Fibre 1g.

Crunchy Fruit Brûlée (v)

This is the quickest ever dessert for a party and an easy treat for the family, especially if your freezer contains a selection of puréed soft fruit.

500g (1lb) any fruit purée (e.g. raspberry, rhubarb, apple, plum, peach, apricot)
150ml (¼pt) low-fat fromage frais
4tsps (4 x 5ml) brown sugar

1. Divide the fruit purée between four ramekin dishes. Pour an equal quantity of fromage frais over each one. Chill in the fridge for at least 2 hours.

2. Sprinkle 1 tsp (1 x 15ml) of brown sugar over each dish, then place under a preheated hot grill until the sugar bubbles and turns golden brown.

3. Chill for at least 2 hours before serving.

Serves: 4

Per portion with apples: Calories 118, Protein 3g, Fat 3g, Carbohydrate 21.5g, Fibre 2.5g; **Per portion with raspberries:** Calories 99, Protein 4g, Fat 3g, Carbohydrate 13g, Fibre 3g;

Per portion with rhubarb: Calories 69, Protein 4g, Fat 3g, Carbohydrate 8g, Fibre 2g.

Pineapple Slices in Red Wine (v)

Pears are often teamed up with red wine, but fresh pineapple cooked in delicious vino tastes even better. Try this with a little low-fat fromage frais or fruit yogurt on top.

1 large ripe pineapple
⅓ bottle (250ml) red wine
2tbsps (2 x 15ml) sugar
small cinnamon stick
4 cloves

1. Peel and slice the pineapple and remove the core with a small sharp knife. Boil the wine, sugar, cinnamon and cloves for 5 minutes.

2. Poach the pineapple slices in the syrup for about 10 minutes. Remove the spices and leave the pineapple to cool in the syrup. Serve in glass dishes.

Serves: 6
Per portion: Calories 90, Protein neg, Fat neg,
Carbohydrate 15g, Fibre 1.2g.

Pavlova (v)

This is a classic Australian dish, which can be adapted according to which soft fruits are in season. Low-fat fromage frais gives the dish a delicious taste and is much lower in calories than double cream.

3 large egg whites
150g (5oz) caster sugar
½tsp (2.5ml) each of vanilla essence and
white wine vinegar
1tsp (5ml) cornflour
300ml (½pt) low-fat fromage frais
200g (7oz) fresh or frozen strawberries,
raspberries or other soft fruit
1 kiwi fruit, peeled and sliced

1. Draw an 18cm (7in) circle on non-stick or rice paper. Place on a baking sheet.
2. Whisk the egg whites until very stiff and whisk in half the sugar. Fold in the remaining sugar, vanilla essence, vinegar and cornflour.
3. Spoon or pipe the mixture on to the paper, to cover the circle. Bake in a preheated oven at 300°F, 150°C, Gas Mark 2 for 15 minutes or until lightly coloured. Reduce the temperature to 250°F, 130°C, Gas Mark ½ for 40–45 minutes. Allow to cool, then remove carefully from the paper. Place on a plate, spoon over the low-fat fromage frais and decorate with fruit.

Serves: 4
Per portion: Calories 267, Protein 8g, Fat 5.5g,
Carbohydrate 49g, Fibre 1g.

Melon Fruit Salad (v)

Spectacular, but very easy to make, this is absolutely delicious. You can either serve it in a large honeydew melon, as suggested in the recipe, or in four small ogen melons.

1 ripe honeydew melon
2 peaches
2 apricots
100g (4oz) strawberries or raspberries
1 apple
1 banana
1tbsp (15ml) lemon juice
2tbsps (2 x 15ml) caster sugar
150ml (¼pt) Madeira wine or port
200g (7oz) seedless white grapes
fresh mint to garnish

1. Slice off one end of the melon, scoop the flesh out of the slice and discard the top. Scoop the seeds out of the rest of the melon and discard.

2. Carefully scoop out the flesh and dice, removing any stray seeds. Cut a zig-zag pattern around the edge of the melon shell.

3. Dip the peaches into hot water, peel and slice. Remove the stones from the apricots and dice the flesh. Hull the strawberries. Mix these fruits together in a large bowl. Core and slice the apple, then peel and slice the banana. Sprinkle both of these fruits with lemon juice. Add the apple and banana to the fruit mixture.

4. Beat the sugar with the wine, pour over the fruit and chill in the refrigerator for 1 hour. Transfer to the melon shell and serve garnished with sprigs of mint.

Serves: 4
Per portion: Calories 197, Protein 2g, Fat neg, Carbohydrate 38g, Fibre 3g.

Spicy Sultana Cheesecake (v)

Everyone loves cheesecake and this one is guaranteed to be popular. It serves up to 8 people, so is a good choice for entertaining.

For the base:
50g (2oz) caster sugar
75g (3oz) low-fat spread
1 medium egg
100g (4oz) self-raising flour
1tsp (2.5ml) each of ground cinnamon and mixed spice

For the cheesecake topping:
200g (7oz) low-fat cottage cheese
200g (7oz) low-fat soft cheese
2 medium eggs, separated
rind and juice of 2 lemons
50g (2oz) caster sugar
2tbsps (2 x 15ml) cornflour
125ml (¼ pt) Shape Double
50g (2oz) sultanas

1. Blend the sugar into the low-fat spread, then beat in the egg, flour and spices. Mix to a soft dough and press out to cover the base of a 20–25cm (8–10in) loose-bottomed cake tin.

2. Beat the cheeses, egg yolks, lemon rind and juice, caster sugar and cornflour together.

3. Whip the Shape Double until it holds its shape and fold into the cheese mixture. Whisk the egg whites until stiff and add to the mixture, with the sultanas. Spoon on to the pastry base.

4. Bake in a preheated oven at 350°F, 180°C, Gas Mark 4 for approximately 1 hour or until the centre is firm to the touch. Should the top begin to colour too much, cover loosely with a piece of greaseproof paper or foil for the remainder of the cooking time. Allow the cheesecake to cool in the tin and then turn out.

Serves: 8
Per portion: Calories 260, Protein 12g, Fat 10g,
Carbohydrate 33g, Fibre 1g.

Figs with Parma Ham
and Sweet Yogurt (v)

Fresh figs are a real treat. Serve this Italian dessert whenever they
are available. It is something very special indeed.

12 fresh figs
280g (10oz) hazelnut-flavour yogurt
3 slices Parma ham, finely shredded

1. Wipe the figs, cut a 3cm (1in) cross into the top of each one with
a sharp knife and squeeze slightly, so they open out to show the
centre of the fruit.
2. Spoon the yogurt over the figs and scatter the Parma ham on
top. Serve chilled.

Serves: 4
Per portion: Calories 141, Protein 7.5g, Fat 3g,
Carbohydrate 23g, Fibre 2.5g.

Further Reading

Here are some further reading suggestions. These are currently published in professional scientific literature. You can order a copy from your local public library.

Janet West and Anne de Looy, 'Sugar wars', *Practice Nurse*,
   21 March 1997

Edited by Richard Cottrell, *Weight Control: The Current
   Perspectives,* Chapman and Hall, 1995

'Sugar free', *Which*, October 1995

T. R. Kirk, S. Burkill and M. Cursiter,'Dietary fat reduction achieved
   by increasing consumption of starchy food', *European Journal
   of Clinical Nutrition*, 1997, Vol 215 455–61

J. P. Flatt, 'Carbohydrate balance and body-weight regulation',
   Proceedings of the Nutrition Society, 1996, Vol 55 449–65

J. Stubbs, 'Dietary macronutrients and glucostatic control of
   feeding', *Proceedings of the Nutrition Society*, 1996, Vol 55
   467–83

A. Astrup and A. Raben, 'Glucostatic control of intake and obesity',
   Proceedings of the Nutrition Society, 1996, Vol 55 495

A. Raben, I. MacDonald and A. Astrup, 'Replacement of dietary fat
   by sucrose and starch: Effects on 14d ad libitum energy intake,
   energy expenditure and body weight in formerly obese and
   never-obese subjects', *International Journal of Obesity*, 1997,
   Vol 21 846–59

Index

Recipes

*Sally and Anne would like to
hear from slimmers who have
tried System S. Please let us
know how the diet worked for
you. Write to us at:*
**System S,
Michael O'Mara Books Ltd,
9 Lion Yard, Tremadoc Road,
London SW4 7NQ**